LAKE VILLA DISTRICT LIBRARY

3 1981 00571 6968

W9-CNC-704

PRAISE FOR *STUNNING SMILES*

Stunning Smiles *looks at oral health as part of our overall health—a critical concept that is missed by most people. It also challenges the readers to look at what they can do and what to avoid to maintain their oral health and develop and maintain a great smile and enhance their confidence. A great read for everyone from an outstanding clinician and compassionate individual who has been through the "dental journey" of being a patient and a provider.*

—ZAHID LALANI, DDS, PHD, MBA

What a gift we have in Dr. Anita Myers' book on dental health and well-being! It is a thorough and engaging look behind the scenes of disease and recovery through the stories of real people. As her colleague and her patient, I can tell you that she puts these concepts into practice every day as she works through treatment options and coaches patients toward better health. Bravo and thanks, Dr. Myers!

—GLENDA OWEN, DDS

It won't take long once you start reading Stunning Smiles *to find that this is way more than just about teeth—it's about total care. Dr. Myers puts it all together in an enjoyable book to help readers get the most out of their smiles. If you are looking for total care, you're in the right place.*

—PHILIP GOLD, CDT

This is a must read! Dr. Myers provides not only a comprehensive overview of what's what in dental care, but also provides great take-away tips and answers to common questions that we all have had. Entertaining, and easy to read, I thank Stunning Smiles *for taking dental care to the next level!*

—SARA STUART, DO

STUNNING SMILES

ANITA MYERS, DDS

stunning
SMILES!

A DENTAL GUIDE TO IMPROVE THE WAY YOU
eat, smile & live

Advantage®

Lake Villa District Library
Lake Villa, Illinois 60046
(847) 356-7711

Copyright © 2018 by Anita Myers.

All rights reserved. No part of this book may be used or reproduced in any manner whatsoever without prior written consent of the author, except as provided by the United States of America copyright law.

Published by Advantage, Charleston, South Carolina.
Member of Advantage Media Group.

ADVANTAGE is a registered trademark, and the Advantage colophon is a trademark of Advantage Media Group, Inc.

Printed in the United States of America.

10 9 8 7 6 5 4 3 2 1

ISBN: 978-1-642250-28-2
LCCN: 2018960314

Book design by Megan Elger.

This publication is designed to provide accurate and authoritative information in regard to the subject matter covered. It is sold with the understanding that the publisher is not engaged in rendering legal, accounting, or other professional services. If legal advice or other expert assistance is required, the services of a competent professional person should be sought.

Advantage Media Group is proud to be a part of the Tree Neutral® program. Tree Neutral offsets the number of trees consumed in the production and printing of this book by taking proactive steps such as planting trees in direct proportion to the number of trees used to print books. To learn more about Tree Neutral, please visit **www.treeneutral.com**.

Advantage Media Group is a publisher of business, self-improvement, and professional development books and online learning. We help entrepreneurs, business leaders, and professionals share their Stories, Passion, and Knowledge to help others Learn & Grow. Do you have a manuscript or book idea that you would like us to consider for publishing? Please visit **advantagefamily.com** or call **1.866.775.1696**.

This book is dedicated to my husband, Brooks, who has unfailingly provided love, support, and encouragement, not only for this project, but also for every aspect of my life.

TABLE OF CONTENTS

PART I: EAT!

PART II: SMILE!

ACKNOWLEDGMENTS

This book began many years ago as a proclamation: "Someday I'm going to write a book about smiles and dental health." The first people to hear this statement were my former team members—Kevin Harberson, Pam Brekeen, Mindy Lang, and Sunshine McLaughlin—who briefly looked a bit stunned and then replied, "Cool!"

In the ensuing years, I rubbed elbows with colleagues and mentors, some of whom had authored books themselves, and they were enthusiastic and encouraging about the idea. I'd like to thank my fellow 3 Knots Study Club members for their spirit about this project: Daren Becker, Irwin Becker, David Bloom, Kelley Brummett, Barbara Devine, Laura Harkin, Ed Mukamal, Ken Myers, Barry Polanski, and Brad Portenoy. I am most grateful to my mentors, Irwin Becker, Donald "Ozzie" Asbjornson, and Rich Green for simultaneously challenging and uplifting me through all my professional endeavors.

My motivation to write this book stalled in 2015 when my husband and I decided to relocate both our home and my practice to a different area of Texas. Once the turmoil subsided, my dear friend and colleague, Jim Lyles, gave new life to the idea. Jim, thank you for all your positive thoughts.

When I proposed the idea of becoming an author to my family, my loving husband, Brooks, was nothing but supportive. My children, Ashley Myers, Blaine Tonking, Heather Holmes, and Reid Tonking also gave their endorsement with energy and excitement. I am so blessed by their love.

I'd also like to express my appreciation and gratitude to my current team members, Debra Henarie and Delma Moreno. Their competence and dedication enabled me to spend additional time on the book and to attend associated meetings. Working with them has been such a pleasure.

Steve Goodman with Advantage Media patiently untangled my words and Lauren Delamater was always just one quick email or call away to make the entire process flow smoothly and calmly. I offer my heartfelt thanks to them and the entire publishing team.

Above all, I'd like to thank my many patients, too numerous to mention by name, for allowing me the privilege of guiding you to a greater level of health. Sharing your lives through this collaborative journey has enriched my existence and fueled my God-given purpose. I am humbled by your friendship and gratitude.

FOREWORD

Over twenty-five years ago, I heard about this exceptional restorative dentist who was just outside of my market area, Dr. Anita. Then twenty-two years ago, I moved my office into a new medical-dental center a few miles away and Dr. Anita had also moved into the same center. She on one end and myself on the other. That way, it was balanced from our modest perspective.

We immediately had great rapport and interaction! Learning the depth and quality of her character was immediate. Then shortly, she was in a divorce, but you would never have known it. Her relationship with her husband, etc. was exceptional! Her approach to relationships was one of being open, empathetic, optimistic, flexible, generous, warm, connected, creative and interesting. Then, I did orthodontic treatment on her younger son. Reid was very high-spirited and highly intelligent, a thoroughbred colt, fun, interesting and a challenge. So, this experience also taught me how exceptional Anita was as a mom.

I have had the honor to work with many exceptional dental professionals over the years. Dental challenges that involve orthodontics excite me. Working with Anita was different. She was able to have a more in-depth perspective: dental, physiological, and emotional. She was never shy about asking for the impossible. At least, what was considered impossible initially. It was amazing how often the totally open communication and synergy resulted in the impossible being accomplished with amazing results. I always knew that when she walked through the door with models in the articulator and she had a determined look, something exciting and beautiful was about to happen. And I knew I was going to be challenged to grow and be innovative for sure!

The creed of one of my primary mentors contained the statement: "Lord, give me a few good friends who know me, yet love me." Anita brings out the best in me as she does for so many others, warts and all. The perpetual student, Anita adds so much value for so many with her dental artistry and with the lives she touches in such a significant way. I am so proud and so honored to be able to call Anita my friend!

Jim Lyles, DDS, orthodontist and owner of Smiles by Lyles in Houston, Texas

INTRODUCTION

Smile and the whole world smiles with you.

Your smile is an amazing work of art and engineering. In health, your smile keeps you well nourished, helps you enjoy social interactions, and plays an integral role in whole-body health. But not all of us are lucky enough to be born with a perfect, winning smile, or we lose this integral connection to physical and emotional health over time, through neglect, disease, or accident. An unhealthy smile can place obstacles in the way of our growth, distract us from our full potential, and limit our accomplishments. We miss the mark of what we want to achieve in life and how we want to express ourselves to others.

Almost everyone has some flaw in their oral health. For some, the flaws are minimal, not even a concern, so that their crooked smile, chipped tooth, or less-than-white teeth become a character trait. As one of my patients who lives in the Texas Hill Country stated, his chipped front tooth made him look "like a real cowboy." But for others, the flaws are devastating, causing them to miss out on opportunities in their careers or relationships, or affecting their overall health, perhaps even contributing to diseases that result in premature death.

I was one of those people with a devastating flaw. When I was fourteen, I was diagnosed with a genetic condition that causes what amounts to premature aging of the mouth and gums, and I was told that I would likely lose all of my teeth by the time I was forty. Since my mom had lost all of her teeth at an early age, that was unacceptable to her. Through struggle and perseverance, she got me to the right kind of oral specialists. I had to have many surgeries and countless other procedures, but when I saw the valiant efforts that all of these dedicated professionals were making just so I could smile and laugh like a normal teenager, I knew I wanted to make that same kind of difference in other people's lives someday, and that is what put me on the path to a career in dentistry.

EAT, SMILE, LIVE

Most people do not understand the critical role their teeth, jaw, and mouth play in their overall health and well-being—that is, until they have a dental problem. For years, the practice of dentistry has been *reactive,* only dealing with a problem once it comes to the surface. This has been the approach of traditional dentistry, and it is a particular problem in the corporate dental world. I want to introduce the reader to a different kind of dentistry, something I like to refer to as lifestyle dentistry, which looks at patients as a whole and seeks to find the *root causes* of their problems rather than just applying a quick fix.

In this book you will meet:

- Paul, a family man, insecure about his own appearance, whose confidence increased after restructuring his smile.

- Tristan, a rebellious teen who refused to follow treatment recommendations but eventually came to realize the important of a healthy smile.

- Donna, a business professional who knew that a better smile could help advance her career, but also came to realize on a personal level that it was the "best decision she ever made."

Their stories, and the stories of countless others, will bring a tear to your eye, maybe a laugh or two, but mostly will teach you how you, too, can have a *Stunning Smile* and improve the way you *Eat, Smile, and Live!*

This is a book for anyone who has ever held their hand over their mouth in a conversation or has never smiled in a family picture. It is to empower them and let them know that it is never too early, or too late, to take control of their dental care.

CHANGING LIVES, ONE SMILE AT A TIME

For many, the opportunity to connect with a smile is lost, or in some cases never really existed. Perhaps a tooth was damaged due to trauma or excessive grinding. Perhaps their teeth have discolored after years of stains from foods and beverages. Or maybe the opportunity for braces in the teen years just wasn't there. The good news is that modern dentistry can solve just about any cosmetic dental problem out there. Dental fears can be managed through simple means, and the cost of most necessary procedures can be financed. I hope this book offers a chance to those who would like to have a healthier, more beautiful smile—and that to those fortunate enough to have a nice smile, it offers the motivation to appreciate its value and make the effort to maintain it—so that all people can enjoy a lifetime of smiles.

Part I

EAT!

*"The food you eat can be either the safest
and most powerful form of medicine
or the slowest form of poison."*

—ANN WIGMORE

CHAPTER 1

YOU ARE WHAT YOU EAT

This is not a book about teeth. It's about food, romance, success and vitality—a little more intriguing, don't you think? It is intended to empower its readers with simple steps to ensure comfort, confidence, and greater overall health.

For instance, imagine you're at a large dinner table with several people. Perhaps it's a holiday meal and everything has been thoughtfully prepared, from appetizers to deserts. Everyone is talking and laughing, simply enjoying each other's company ... except one person who isn't smiling or laughing because she simply feels self-conscious about her smile and makes a conscious effort to conceal it. Then there's a guy who must not care for the food; he barely picks at his meal and avoids anything chewy or crunchy, which includes just about everything from the salad through dessert. You and the others don't realize how uncomfortable it is for him to chew, because an annoying tooth pain just won't go away.

Eating and smiling are intimately related in a kind of vicious cycle. Eating the wrong foods—too much sugar and poor nutrition—can significantly damage your dental health, which in turn can affect your overall health, and dental problems that do not allow you to eat and enjoy your food leave you with very little to smile about.

PAUL'S STORY

Except in the case of dental emergencies, I take several photos of each patient's smile as part of their initial examination. This is a process I could delegate to an assistant, but I take these pictures myself because I feel it's important that I understand each patient's perception of their own smile. Many people hide their teeth when they smile, barely curving their lips or showing any enamel. However, they do not realize that they come across to others as sad or pained, reluctant, or unengaged by smiling this way. Is that really how they want to be perceived by their friends and family?

Earlier in my career, I met Paul, who was very self-conscious about his smile and made great efforts to hide it. He was a devoted father and successful businessman, friendly with everyone he met, but he almost never smiled. In his initial visit, in order to evaluate his "smile reveal" and determine what cosmetic dentistry procedures would give him the confidence to smile more, I asked him to smile for the camera. His lips barely moved. In an attempt to get him to smile bigger for these photos, I asked him to say "eeee ..." He kind of grimaced, still barely showing any of his teeth.

Based on his limited expressions, he and I determined that we would not have to address the appearance of the teeth in the back of his mouth; his old crowns were sufficient and would never show anyway—or so we thought. After a treatment plan that focused on restoring his front teeth was completed, Paul changed. He became more confident, more outgoing, and was more engaging in conversations with others. His smile stretched wide and literally lit up the room. Initially, I was disappointed that we didn't include those "hidden" back teeth in the treatment plan so that the final result would be even better. But Paul was happy, and I realized that was what really mattered.

THE SWEET TOOTH

It is not only normal for humans to crave sweets, it is in our DNA.[1] Babies are born with an innate craving for sugar and carbohydrates—because sugar and carbohydrates mean energy, and infants need energy to grow. From an evolutionary and anthropological perspective, three square meals a day were not always on the menu for our hunter-gatherer ancestors, so there was an evolutionary imperative to be drawn to foods that were sweet, to load up on needed calories. Finding enough calories to make it through your day may not be a problem for most of us anymore, but that genetic desire for sugar remains.

Now let me be clear: Sugar by itself doesn't cause cavities. There also has to be a susceptible host, a specific kind of bacteria, and a certain amount of time for this "perfect storm" of events to occur that leads to tooth decay. But since we can't control most of these components, and we can increase our awareness about our sugar consumption, let's take a closer look at the sweetness factor.

---

1   D.R. Reed and A.H. McDaniel, "The Human Sweet Tooth." *BMC Oral Health* 6, suppl. 1 (2006), https://doi.org/10.1186/1472-6831-6-S1-S17.

Lots of foods, especially processed foods, have added sugars. Take smoothies, for example. With smoothies, you think you're eating something healthy, but they often have high levels of added sugar. Yogurt is another one people get tripped up on. If left alone, yogurt can be very healthy, and some are, but others are ridiculously sweetened, to the level of candy or breakfast cereals.

There are also many different kinds of sugar in our food, but it is common table sugar, or sucrose, that is top of the list at promoting the production of acid that causes cavities. Not that the other ones can't cause cavities, but the bacteria that promote tooth decay have a "sweet tooth" of their own, and they prefer sucrose because it makes for a better growth medium.

While sucrose may be the biggest offender, other kinds of sugar also cause problems. This is where a lot of people get into trouble, because while sweet things such as honey and agave syrup have slight nutritional benefits over table sugar, they are almost as bad for you when it comes to tooth decay. Beware of corn syrup and corn syrup solids, and the ubiquitous high fructose corn syrup, which is a term food manufacturers came up with to sneak sugar into processed foods.

Ingredients that are often paired with sugar, like refined white flour, are among the worst of the worst. For example, if you eat a cupcake, you are getting a double whammy from the sugar and that starchy carbohydrate in the flour, and that combination provides a more attractive environment to the bacteria that cause cavities.

If you look at the labels, sugar is usually identified in grams. There are about four grams of sugar per teaspoon. Not that anyone pays much attention to serving size, which is another problem entirely, but when you look at a serving of breakfast cereal and it's got eleven or sixteen grams of sugar, you're looking at three to four teaspoons per serving. Would you ever take an unsweetened cereal and dump four teaspoons of sugar into it? But that is what the food company already put in there for you, and as I said, most people ignore the serving size and double- or triple-dose themselves or their kids on sugar.

One thing that people tend to overlook is that it is not only the volume of sugar that you ingest that can be problematic for teeth, it is the length of time of exposure. This is why sticky foods that contain sugar, such as Tootsie Rolls or gummy bears, are a worse choice if you must grab a piece of candy, or even things like Lifesavers, which you keep in your mouth and suck on for a long time. I tell patients it's not about the quantity of sugar as much as it is about their exposures to sugar. Let's say you have a twin brother and you both like coffee. You get up in the morning and put ten spoons of sugar in your coffee cup, and that one cup is the only one you drink all day. You would have approximately twenty minutes of acid exposure in your mouth after consuming that coffee. In contrast, your brother takes only one spoon of sugar with each cup, but he has ten cups a day. With twenty minutes for each exposure, he has two hundred minutes exposure per day compared to your twenty, even though you both consumed the same amount. He's probably going to have more cavities than you.

I had one female patient, let's call her Pattie. Pattie had been seeing me for years, she always had a good checkup, and she was really diligent about her six-month cleanings. But one time she came in and I was floored to see that she had fourteen cavities. I couldn't believe it, so I had to try and deduce what changed. What had occurred to cause such a radical shift in her dental health? She denied that she was eating anything sweet and said she had not changed her diet at all since her last visit. But then she told me she had recently gotten a new job as a receptionist, and she was concerned that in speaking to the public, she would have bad breath, so she was popping Tic-Tacs all day long, every day. That was chronic sugar exposure taking its toll, from something as small and seemingly insignificant as a Tic-Tac.

THE SUGAR IMPOSTERS

Even when you want to avoid sugar, it can be harder than you think. Sugar is in everything—it's in ketchup, salad dressings, soup, and bread. And food makers do a very good job of hiding sugar in their products with names of ingredients that you may not immediately recognize as sugar. I call these the "sugar imposters." Some of the most popular of these to be on the lookout for are:

- Anhydrous dextrose
- Brown sugar
- Cane crystals
- Cane sugar
- Corn sweetener
- Corn syrup
- Corn syrup solids
- Crystal dextrose
- Evaporated cane juice
- Fructose sweetener
- Fruit juice concentrates
- High fructose corn syrup
- Liquid fructose
- Malt syrup
- Maple syrup
- Molasses

- Pancake syrup
- Raw sugar

OVERCOMING THE CRAVING FOR SWEETS

There is no getting around the natural imperative to crave sweets, but you can tame your taste buds with some wiser choices. You can choose fruit when you want brownies, nibble some stevia-sweetened chocolate when you can't get the thought of candy out of your head, and gradually fill your cup with less sweet tea and more unsweet tea until it's totally unsweet. Parents can take a more proactive role in minimizing the development of the proverbial sweet tooth in our kids. Parents do the shopping, so it's up to us. We can make better choices about what we put in our grocery cart once we know how.

It is up to us as loving parents to teach kids about making healthier food choices. I think we should teach kids at a very early age what real food is—what it looks like and where it comes from—so that they not only minimize their taste for sweets but also know how to recognize and make good food choices. I suggest that parents tell their kids to look around at what they see growing on trees: apples and bananas, or Snickers bars and Twinkies? What do they see flowing in our streams and rivers: Hi-C and Coca-Cola, or crisp, pure water? Food that comes from nature is what we were meant to eat. Another revealing observation is in how you feel after eating certain foods. How do you feel after eating an apple? Compare that to how you feel after eating a doughnut (or two).

We need to find ways to make healthy foods as colorful and appealing as the candy and breakfast cereals. Be creative! One thing I did with my own kids was to cut oranges into attractive slices and cut grapes into small bunches, and lay those out on platters in the fridge with some slices of cheese, so that it looked nice and tantalizing when they opened the refrigerator door, and they could just pop what they liked into their mouths.

Think about providing other kinds of healthy options, such as sliced carrots and celery sticks with hummus to dip them in. You do not have to cut out the muffins and cookies entirely, but save them for once in a while, or special occasions, and your kids will not develop a need or expectation for them every single day.

ARTIFICIAL SWEETENERS AND SUGAR SUBSTITUTES

You might think that sugar substitutes are a better bet for your teeth than sugar. To a degree, that may be true. Sugar substitutes are considered any sweetener you may consume that isn't table sugar. These substitutes include:

- Artificial sweeteners

- Sugar alcohols

- Novel sweeteners (such as stevia)

- Natural sweeteners like honey, molasses, and agave nectar

For example, if you are going to suck on a hard candy, a sugar-free one is probably better than a regular one. There is one sugar alcohol, xylitol, which in some studies was shown to actually prevent cavities.[2] However, given the other known negative impacts on health of most sugar substitutes, they are still best used sparingly. These substitutes are often not even effective for weight loss. Many times people trying to lose weight wind up making up for the calories they think they are saving with diet sodas and other sugar-free treats by overindulging on

---

2   P.A. Nayak, U.A. Nayak, and V. Khandelwal, "The Effect of Xylitol on Dental Caries and Oral Flora," *Clinical, Cosmetic and Investigational Dentistry* 6 (2014): 89–94. https://doi.org/10.2147/CCIDE.S55761.

other foods. There is also a theory that suggests that these artificial sweeteners trick our bodies and interfere with the way we process foods. Our brains are wired to associate sweetness with high calories. When we eat something that is artificially sweetened that does not also have the concurrent calories to metabolize, it throws off everything—from digestion to our taste buds.

RETHINK WHAT YOU DRINK

A majority of kids and almost half of the adults in the United States drink at least one sugar-sweetened beverage every day.[3] One of my patients is a high school football player who admitted he drinks an average of ten sugary sodas or sports beverages a day. While most people know drinking sugary drinks can cause cavities, they may not realize that another cause of decay is dental erosion, which happens when teeth are exposed to the acids found in sweet beverages, fruit juices, and diet sodas.

IT'S NOT JUST SUGAR

Even though many of us overindulge in it, we all kind of know that sugar is bad for our teeth. But there are also many other foods that can cause dental issues. For example, I had three people in my office one day, in three different rooms, and it was such a coincidence that all three had damaged a tooth on a popcorn kernel. One of them chipped a tooth, but I was able to polish it and it was fine. One of them broke a tooth a little bit, but I was able to fill it. The third one broke a tooth so badly that it split in half and had to be removed.

---

3 "Get the Facts: Sugar-Sweetened Beverages and Consumption," Centers for Disease Control and Prevention website, last updated April 7, 2017, https://www.cdc.gov/nutrition/data-statistics/sugar-sweetened-beverages-intake.html.

We are omnivores, and our dentition is designed for both grinding and shredding. Our teeth are perfectly fine for almonds, peanuts, hazelnuts, and the like, but very hard things, such as corn nuts and popcorn kernels, can cause problems for our teeth.

If you have jaw issues, such as TMJ, you want to avoid chewy, hard things like beef jerky or any kind of tough meat, or doughy things such as pizza crust or bagels—anything that can cause you to overwork your jaw.

THE DENTAL DIET

If you really think about it, the diet that is best for your teeth and oral health is the same one that is best for your overall health. Do you want to eat the best foods for a healthy smile? Stick with anything that comes off of a plant: broccoli, cauliflower, lettuce, tomatoes, peppers, avocados, etc. Like your mom always said, minimize the sweets and eat your vegetables. Beyond that, eggs and meats, nuts, whole grains, and fish high in omega-3 fatty acids, such as tuna, salmon, and sardines, should all be part of your dental diet. Basically, anything that hasn't been adulterated by man and tagged with a label is going to be good for your teeth.

EAT THIS, NOT THAT

You can make different, healthier choices for your teeth and your body throughout the day. What do most people eat when they get up in the morning? Do you go to Starbucks or Dunkin' Donuts and get a croissant, muffin, or doughnut and a coffee loaded with sugar? Instead, maybe give yourself some more time to grab a bowl of whole grain cereal at home. You could sweeten it with fruit or a sugar substitute like stevia. Or have an egg, or better yet, egg whites with spinach. If you have no time to cook, make yourself a protein shake. Most have very little sugar in them, like one gram. Add some fruit for a homemade low-sugar smoothie, instead of the smoothies with added sugar sold in most shops and drive-throughs.

For lunch, instead of having a sandwich with bread and a side of fries and a soft drink, try making a wrap. My dental assistant, Delma, uses collard leaves or Swiss chard, and lays her ingredients out on that. For example, take a slice of Swiss cheese and some roasted turkey, or some sort of lunch meat, and all the veggies that you like, and then roll it up and eat it like a burrito. You will find some more "eat this, not that" options at the end of this chapter.

EAT FOR LIFE!

The fact that, for the most part, the foods that are best eaten and avoided for good oral health align very closely with those for overall health is a reflection of the profound link between a healthy smile and a healthy life. Since dentistry and general medicine have long been distinct practices, most people tend to separate the mouth from the rest of the body. If there's a diet that's good for your left arm, we all realize that it will be good for your right arm as well. The same goes for your mouth. If you eat a diet that's good for your mouth, it only stands to reason that it will be good for all of your organs. There is current evidence that the common denominator in many health issues, including heart disease, diabetes, Alzheimer's disease, and even some cancers, is inflammation.[4] A diet that is rich in non-inflammatory foods and that promotes a healthy balance of good bacteria versus bad bacteria in the gut is ideal for a healthy mouth

---

4   Y.Z. Liu, Y.X. Wang, and C.L. Jiang. "Inflammation: The Common Pathway of Stress-Related Diseases," *Frontiers in Human Neuroscience* 11 (2017): 316, https://doi.org/10.3389/fnhum.2017.00316.

as well as longevity. Inflammation is part of your body's immune response. Processed and other unnatural foods, as well as excess sugar, can put your body's immune system on overdrive, resulting in a chronic state of inflammation.

It's all connected. Here's an example: If you are eating poorly, it can throw off your digestive system, and that can lead to acid reflux. The acid reflux has the potential to prevent you from getting a good night's sleep, because that acid causes inflammation in the back of the throat, behind the nose, which can lead to sleep apnea, which can lead to any number of problems related to sleep deprivation. Beyond that, the regurgitated acid is corrosive and damaging to the teeth and esophagus.

I've had some cases where people are facing major restorations because of the erosion from the acid that is the result of GERD (gastroesophageal reflux disease, or acid reflux).

It's all a matter of balance and making the right choices. For example, I tell patients we have to accept the fact that sugar exists. It is in our foods and it's a part of our lives, but we have the power to control it and not let it control us. Balance and moderation are the key. You need to make sweets an occasional treat rather than the routine habit they have become for many. Balance in nutrition helps your brain, your heart, your liver, your lungs, your kidneys, everything—eating right can put a smile on your face in more ways than one.

TIPS AND TAKEAWAYS

Sugar-Free Recipes

- Simply substitute the sugar in any recipe with non-GMO erythritol. It is a natural sugar alcohol that has essentially zero calories, doesn't affect blood sugar, and doesn't cause tooth decay. Unlike most sugar alcohols, 90 percent of it is absorbed unchanged in the small intestine and excreted in the urine, meaning it has a low incidence of bowel irritation like some other sugar alcohols. It looks like table sugar and measures like table sugar, but it's rated as 70 percent of the sweetness of cane sugar. (Since I don't care for super-sweetness, I find this to be an advantage for most recipes.) It can be combined with a small amount of maple extract (3/4 tsp per cup of erythritol) to create a substitute for brown sugar. To minimize exposure to health risks, it's important to specify non-GMO brands of erythritol, which I buy from Amazon.[5]

- The other sweetener I use is stevia. I use a small packet of the powdered form to sweeten tea or lemonade and I use stevia drops along with erythritol for cooking if I want a sweeter result. I find stevia to have a pleasant, sweet taste, although some people feel that it has a bitter aftertaste. Stevia is available in any grocery store on the sugar/baking aisle.

- Keep in mind that dental decay comes from (1) production of acid by bacteria due to (2) exposure to "fermentable carbohydrates"—not just sugar—in (3) a susceptible host over (4) a period of time. Substituting sugar in a cookie recipe doesn't eliminate all fermentable carbohydrates, such as flour … and chips and crackers can promote decay as well.

- Apples are sweet due to fructose, which theoretically can be metabolized by bacteria in the mouth, but sucrose is much more easily metabolized and is more likely to cause cavities in the teeth. Apples are considered a "detergent food," which means the texture of the food actually scrubs the teeth while chewing, thereby minimizing the incidence of decay.

Food Presentation

- It's easier to encourage children to eat decay-resistant foods if those foods are appealing to the eyes. A simple solution is to simply peel and cut fruits, cheese, and vegetables ahead of time and store them in the refrigerator, ready to eat. If cutting apple slices, dip them in water with a little lemon juice added to keep them from turning brown.

- Check out Pinterest.com and search for "fun food for kids" for a host of great ideas on food presentation.

BETTER DIET CHOICES

Breakfast

INSTEAD OF	TRY
White bread	Seed bread
Jelly on toast	Avocado on toasted seed bread
Peanut butter and jelly	Peanut butter and apple slices
Breakfast pastry or doughnut	Chai spice mug cake*
Egg biscuit sandwich	Egg poached on mild salsa
Boxed cereal	Whole oats (with stevia)
Pancakes with syrup	Whole grain pancakes with sugar-free syrup
Orange juice (four oranges = 8 oz)	One orange

*   https://www.ruled.me/chai-spice-keto-mug-cake/

Lunch and Dinner

INSTEAD OF	TRY
Sandwich	Lettuce wrap with meat/cheese/veggie filling
Canned soup	Homemade soup with broth base
Hamburger	"Burger" salad
Chicken enchiladas	Lite chicken tacos
Spaghetti and sauce	Spaghetti squash and sauce

Beverages

INSTEAD OF	TRY
Soda	Water
Lemonade	Water with a squeeze of lemon and stevia
Fruit drinks	Water with a sugar-free flavor enhancer
Sugar-sweetened tea and coffee	Unsweetened or stevia-sweetened tea and coffee

CHAPTER 2

THE TOOTH, THE WHOLE TOOTH, AND NOTHING BUT THE TOOTH!

JIM'S STORY

Jim was the general manager of a major hotel in a large metropolitan area. His dedication to his work required long hours, short weekends, and few vacations. "Frankly," he told me, "I haven't had time to take care of myself." His "reactive" —rather than "proactive" —approach to dental health resulted in the loss of many of his teeth, to the point that it was extremely difficult for him to eat, speak, or even smile. Part of his reluctance to save his smile was that his parents had both lost their teeth at an early age, so he just assumed he was destined to suffer the same fate. Fortunately, we were able to restore many of Jim's teeth and replace the ones he lost. Jim was extremely grateful to be able once again to eat comfortably and smile without embarrassment.

Jim is not alone. Too many of us are like Jim—so involved in our busy lives that dental care, and indeed all health care, takes a back seat, and we only go to see the doctor or dentist when we have a problem.

A STITCH IN TIME ...

I'm sure you are familiar with the old adage "A stitch in time saves nine." This proverb really has nothing to do with stitches, or the fabric of reality, but rather with the very real-world lesson that putting in a little time on something now can save you a whole lot more time in the future. This is another problem I often run into with patients who feel they simply do not have the time to devote to their dental care.

I had one patient, Terry, who worked for an offshore oil company, and from the sound of it, she had a very, very busy schedule. During the week, it was practically impossible for her to get off any time from work, and I think that was a good part of the reason she let a problem with some older dental work go on for so long. She had a crown on a bottom left tooth that had not been properly fitted from the outset. It was too tall and too wide, so every time Terry bit together, she'd hit there first. And because she was so busy at work and because nobody likes to go to the dentist anyway, she just put up with it for the longest time. By the time she came to see me—I think it had been about three years—the tooth below the crown had become severely infected and the nerves had died. It looked like the tooth could not be saved. But we were able to take off the ill-fitting crown, perform root canal therapy and replace the bad crown with a comfortable temporary. She was able to wear that temporary for quite a few months until everything was healed, and even the temporary had her doing so much better than the discomfort she went through for years with that horribly ill-fitting crown.

At first, I thought financial difficulties must be the reason someone would put up with that misaligned bite and not return to the dentist who'd originally done the work and have it fixed. However, Terry explained that she felt it was worth it at that time to muddle through for months, and then years, rather than lose the day or two at work it would have taken to repair and replace the original crown. When she came to me, we removed the old crown, repaired the tooth, and eventually got her a proper fitting crown to align with the rest of her bite. But all of that took more visits, and was far costlier, than had she taken the time to address the problem early on. Had she done that, she might have avoided the need for the root canal. So Terry worried about missing time at work, but in the long run, she had to take more days off from the job—a perfect example of "a stitch in time" and the value of addressing any dental problems as soon as they arise. The moral of the story is that when it comes to dental care, a proactive approach can save time, money, and aggravation.

TO SAVE THE TOOTH

We really got lucky in Terry's case. Had she gone on just a bit longer, I do not know if we would have been able to save her tooth. Ultimately, no matter what has caused damage to your teeth—disease, decay, or injury—that is always our goal, to save the natural teeth. Sometimes this can be another problem where patients can get lazy about being proactive, because in reality, they may not share that goal. It is wonderful that as a modern dental practitioner I have all of these tools at my disposal to repair, restore, and now—with implants—replace your teeth if necessary. But assuming your teeth don't have developmental problems, there is nothing—no crown, bridge, denture, or implant—that is as good as your own natural teeth. Sometimes having all of this great dental technology at our disposal can be a bit of a double-edged sword. Patients will often let things go because they have the mistaken impression that it does not really matter because dentists can fix that, no problem. However, any dentist, and especially in my practice, would rather teach you how to *prevent* losing your teeth than put you through having them restored or replaced. A lot of this stems from the fact that for some reason, people simply do not think of their teeth the same way they do the rest of their body. Most of us would not purposefully engage in behaviors that would risk losing a finger, an arm, or a leg, and yet many do not think twice about behaviors that put their teeth at risk. When you marvel at a new baby and look down at his or her tiny wiggly ten fingers and ten toes, and cute little nose and all that, you realize how perfect we are just the way we are. Imagine how horrible it would be for that baby to lose a finger, a hand, or an ear. Yet I find that most people do not make that association with teeth. They think: *Well, if I lose my teeth, it's no big deal. I'll just get some new teeth.* Now, it is true that if, heaven forbid, you lose a leg, you can get a prosthetic leg, but at this point in time, that artificial leg will never work as well as the real one. People need to come to that same realization with teeth. Yes, we can replace your teeth if that becomes absolutely necessary, but as a general rule natural, healthy teeth are superior to man-made replacements.

THE MOST COMMON CAUSES OF TOOTH LOSS

While it is always my goal to prevent tooth loss, unfortunately there are times when that is not possible. Injuries, and particularly sports injuries, are among the most common causes of a tooth damaged beyond repair. Any kind of sports-related injuries can be a problem; I've had cases involving diving off a diving board, falling off a bicycle, running into somebody's elbow on a football or baseball field, and getting hit in the face with a ball in competitive sports. And it is not just injuries from sports—fist fights, slip and falls, car wrecks, and accidents with tools can all damage or knock out teeth. One of my patients was at the drive-up window at her bank. She thought she'd rolled the window down, but the window had only gone down a little way, and she turned her head and chipped a tooth on the partially rolled down window.

With these kinds of injuries, the nature of the repair depends on the extent of the damage. Again, our goal is always to save the tooth whenever possible. Did you know that if you or your child gets a permanent tooth knocked out, you can possibly save the tooth if you can stick it back in there? If it's dirty, you dip it in milk, or in water if you don't have milk, and then position it back in the socket immediately. Be sure you DON'T scrub the tooth—the fibers on the root are necessary for reattachment. Then get to your dentist as quickly as possible. The tooth might end up with a root canal in the future, but a lot of times the ligaments that hold the tooth to the socket will heal, and a little quick-thinking dental first aid may mean the difference between keeping that tooth or not. If the tooth does have to be removed, we can replace it with an implant, which is the current state of the art for tooth replacement, or with other tooth-replacement options.

Sports injuries, particularly in kids, may be some of the most common causes of tooth loss, but they are certainly not the only ones. In fact, sometimes tooth loss can be caused by something a lot less obvious and subtler than a jaw meeting the sidewalk or a diving board.

As we have mentioned before, not being proactive, poor home care, and/or poor diet, along with susceptibility issues, can lead to problems, particularly gum disease and bone loss around the teeth. The typical scenario is where we would lose the multi-rooted teeth first, starting with the upper teeth in the back. Then the lower molars are lost, and before long, it becomes very difficult to chew. People don't realize what happens because it's so gradual, and there's seldom any pain until the late stages of the disease.

Three out of four adults in America suffer from some form of gum disease—mild, moderate, or advanced. As the gums become inflamed, the bone recedes, the teeth loosen, and eventually teeth begin to fall out.

This kind of gradual tooth loss is actually a little bit harder to strategize. If you're going to replace one tooth now, then what about the rest of them? We need to develop a plan for the long term. Many practitioners will take this as a battle-by-battle strategy, replacing teeth as they fall out without a real plan to win the war. I try to take a more proactive and comprehensive approach, and with the help of a gum specialist (called a periodontist), we can bring in techniques such as laser therapy, more frequent cleanings, and/or gum surgery if necessary. This way, we do our best to get gum recession under control and give patients the tools that they need at home to maintain healthier gums on a daily basis, do everything they can to support their immune system, fight the good fight, and prevent further tooth loss.

Poor oral hygiene, gum disease, and sports injuries can all lead to tooth loss, but of all the possible reasons for tooth loss, one of the most gut-wrenching causes, which we see all too often, is domestic abuse.

ROSEMARY'S STORY

Three missing front teeth did nothing to help Rosemary's appearance. So she quit trying to look nice, quit going out to meet other people, even quit her job. She stayed at home, watched the rest of the world on television, and hid from a society that would judge and perhaps ridicule her.

In 1977, she was a pretty young woman, full of life, when she met the man she thought she wanted to be with forever. But some marriages go through a mysterious, awful change after the wedding, and this was the case for Rosemary. For more than twenty years, she endured domestic abuse and never reported it. The emotional abuse started in the first few years after her marriage, but by then, she'd already had children and wanted to keep her family together, so like many women, she suffered in silence. Gradually, over the course of her marriage, what started as emotional abuse escalated to violence and physical abuse—but still, Rosemary felt she could endure a bad marriage for the sake of her family. She still harbored a secret hope, somewhere deep inside, that her husband would one day abandon the drugs and alcohol that brought out his angry side and return again to the man she once adored. But alas, her hopes were in vain, and instead he moved on to abusing stronger and more dangerous drugs. Sometime after their twenty-fifth wedding anniversary, engulfed in a rage brought on by crack cocaine, he began slapping her, then punching her in the face and chest and kicking her in the legs and torso. In addition to multiple bruises and lacerations, his blows knocked out three of her front teeth, fractured another, and caused hemorrhaging in one eye.

After such a violent attack, Rosemary finally got the help she needed to break free of her husband and the demons that bound her to him. After the divorce, she underwent counseling at a nearby women's center, where she heard about the American Academy of Cosmetic Dentistry's Give Back a Smile (GBAS) program. Even though she didn't drive a car, she was willing to arrange transportation out of town, or even out of state if necessary, to find a dentist willing to help.

That dentist just happened to be me. I'll be honest—I struggled with the notion of volunteering my time and materials to participate in the GBAS program. At that moment, I didn't really consider the fact that my lab technicians would donate their skills and materials. I thought I would bear that expense as well. Like the cartoon character with a devil on one shoulder and an angel on the other, I weighed the pros and cons. Perhaps it was divine intervention, or maybe the emotional factors outweighing the logical ones, but finally, the angel won. That little voice in the back of my mind reminded me that I was truly blessed and that I had been given talents and skills that would help others less fortunate. So I volunteered and waited to hear from the AACD.

When Rosemary first came to my office, she was reserved, shy, and rather plain. Her worn clothes and lack of makeup didn't help the fact that she refused to smile or even to talk much. She avoided eye contact and looked down at her lap much of the time. But she cooperated in every way possible. She was so eager to help us as we took radiographs and impressions.

A few weeks later, the work began. After a five-hour appointment, she had a new upper arch and a new smile. Something clicked inside Rosemary that day as she looked into the mirror. I like to think she recognized the woman that she used to be and could become again. By the time her case was completed, Rosemary had blossomed. Her hair had been styled, she wore makeup, and she smiled constantly. She had tears in her eyes as she hugged me good-bye and thanked me for giving her smile back. I had tears in my eyes, too.

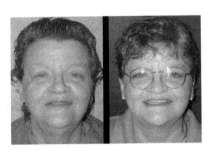

In a card she later sent, she wrote, "Words or actions cannot express how much I appreciate all you have done for me. Every time I look in the mirror and smile, I will always think of you and what you did for me. My outlook on life has changed dramatically for the good. To take time out of your busy schedule to help me, meant more to me than you will ever know. Thanks go to you and your staff for all the kindness and respect they showed me."

Yes, Rosemary received her smile and all the benefits that confidence brings into a person's life. But Rosemary gave me a gift as well. By receiving with gratitude and appreciation, she let me experience giving, and that warm sense of fulfillment that only comes with sharing and caring for another individual.

EASING FEAR AND RELIEVING GUILT

It takes a lot of courage for someone as abused as Rosemary to come forward and get help, but things do not have to be so extreme for people to fear coming to the dentist. I know that often people realize that they have caused their own problems by eating too many sweets, skipping dental cleanings, and otherwise not taking those proactive dental health steps we've been speaking about. This can lead to a kind of guilt and embarrassment that prevents them from coming in to get the work that they need—even when they know they have a dental problem—because they are afraid they will be lectured by the dentist. People need to know that this is a wrong way of thinking, especially in my practice. I will never make a patient feel bad for the condition of their mouth. In my mind, why you got to the point you did is far less important than the fact that you are now here for help. Of course, eventually we will get into the root causes of why the patient wound up with the presenting problem, but especially on that first visit, it is all about assuaging fears and building trust.

We do that by always trying to find something positive to remark on. Usually it starts with the X-rays. We take a panoramic X-ray. If we can't get one from a previous office, we'll take a new one here, and I'll point out, "I see no signs of oral cancer. Your jaw joints look good and sound. I don't see any degenerative changes there. You've got good bone level. Here's a root canal from a long time ago and it seems to be intact." So they get a little bit of positive reinforcement at first, an "attaboy" before they even go into the room with the dental chair.

One of the other things we do in that first visit is try to give the patients tips and tricks to take home. I'll tell them, "If you come here twice a year to get your teeth cleaned, who's going to be in charge for the other 363 days a year? I want to be your coach, your advocate, so that you have the tools you need to take care of your mouth in a way that promotes good oral health." This is because I find that nobody's ever really told them what they need to be doing to be more proactive.

We use a pink coloring agent on several of the teeth to show them the nature of the bacteria that causes problems. When I do this, I'll try to point out what they are doing right in terms of brushing and what they can work on to get an even better result. "Look, right here there's no pink stain remaining. You're doing a really good job here. If you want to crank it up a little bit, here's where the bacteria are hiding from you, and this is the tool that you need to use to get in that area."

They typically leave saying, "That was fun. I didn't expect to have a good time at the dentist or feel like I made friends." It's a positive experience for everybody. And I think they do leave with more information. I tell them they need to stop calling their toothbrush a toothbrush because in reality, it is a gum massager. Most people were just handed a toothbrush by their parents when they were about two or three years old and told to brush their teeth, but few of us were actually taught the proper way to brush from an early age.

So that is why I tell them this is not a toothbrush, it's a gum massager. I don't want them to simply put it on the top of their teeth, I want them to put it at about a forty-five degree angle to the gum and gently massage. Now they're going to get 100 percent of that tooth surface clean. They're going to stimulate circulation in the gum, and they're going to eliminate the bacteria. Then they need to get either a pick or floss in between the teeth where the brush can't reach.

We talk about Waterpiks, ultrasonic toothbrushes, toothpaste brands, fluoride or no fluoride, what kind of mouth rinse to use, and more. There's a lot of information that I make sure they take home, so they feel empowered after that first visit, and almost 100 percent of the time, I hear things such as "Wow, I have never had a dental visit like that before."

TIPS AND TAKEAWAYS

- Being proactive and addressing small problems when they first occur will prevent bigger problems later on.

- Not taking the time to address dental problems when they first occur will lead to more costly repairs that take more time to complete.

- You can possibly save a permanent tooth that has been knocked out, by rinsing it in milk or water and sticking it back in the socket.

- You should think of your toothbrush as more of gum massager, and always brush at a forty-five degree angle to the teeth.

- You should never feel too embarrassed, afraid, or guilty regarding a dental problem to see your dentist.

CHAPTER 3

THE ROOT OF THE PROBLEM

All too often, dental treatment is recommended in response to a specific problem. For instance, if someone breaks a tooth, they get a crown; if they have a cavity, they get a filling. We need to look beyond the obvious and ask *why* the tooth broke, *why* the patient got a cavity. Maybe there's a bite problem that caused the tooth to break and if we don't address that, another tooth is likely to break in the near future. Perhaps the cavity was caused by a food trap, which was the result of tooth movement. If we don't deduce *why* the tooth moved, the same problem can continue to occur in other areas of the mouth.

I like to say that what we practice is something called lifestyle dentistry. Maybe a better term would be relationship dentistry, because basically, it is a relationship-based practice where I spend quite a bit of time, especially during the first visit, getting to know the patient. That means not only getting to know the patients' mouths, but getting to know a lot about them as people—their habits, their hobbies, what they do for a living, their lifestyle—because all of these things are going to factor into the root causes of any dental issues, and will help us work better together to bridge the gap (pardon the pun) between where they are now and where they should be in terms of oral health.

It means looking beyond the surface. For example, if I am doing an initial examination and I see an obvious crack in a tooth, my dental brain instantly thinks that it is going to need a crown. But if the person behind the tooth has other issues going on, perhaps that might not be the correct immediate course of action. Let's say she has three kids in college, and on top of that she's going through breast cancer treatments. Then I feel it is my job to see what I can do to maybe bypass some of the more time-consuming forms of traditional dentistry, to get her to a place where she can prioritize her needs and put dentistry in an appropriate category.

Here is one that is not hypothetical. I once had an elderly gentleman who was not in good health, and he came to me knowing that he would soon need to be hospitalized to care for his other health issues. On top of his otherwise degrading health, he had been procrastinating about getting a severely decayed tooth treated. When I saw him, we removed the tooth right away, knowing that he was on the verge of a hospital stay. Had I not known of his impending hospitalization, I might have taken less aggressive measures to treat his tooth. However, knowing that the last thing you want to experience while lying in a hospital bed is a severe toothache, having to contend with that constant throbbing and aching on top of trying to deal with other issues, that was the right course of action.

These are just a few examples, but it is the same with every patient. When I can get to know more about the person's lifestyle and habits, and some of their unique circumstances and wishes, it helps me to better coordinate an individualized treatment plan tailored specifically for them.

HOWARD'S STORY

There's never a convenient time for a tooth to break. Even if there's no discomfort involved, the social awkwardness of being in public with a missing front tooth, or the difficulty of chewing when a tooth cracks or crown comes off—even in an unseen rear tooth—is at best an unwelcome annoyance.

Howard had old crowns, or caps, on most of his teeth. The first time one in front broke off, he didn't think it was much of a problem—there was no pain involved, because the tooth below the crown had already had a root canal, so Howard went to his dentist and merely had it re-cemented.

Howard was a businessman with a very busy schedule. He traveled extensively meeting with clients. When another front crown broke off, again he was not in pain, and this time he did not want to take the time to see his dentist and tried to put it back in place himself using over-the-counter dental cement. But the crown would wiggle every time he tried to chew and eventually came out again. The crowns on both of these teeth continued to come loose and break off. Eventually, it got to the point where Howard's dentist could not reseat the crowns, and he recommended he have the two teeth pulled and replaced with dental implants.

While dental implants are a reliable way to replace missing or hopeless teeth, Howard's problem wasn't that his teeth were hopeless. His current dentist was failing to address the root of the problem, which was that his bite was off and he was grinding excessively in the areas that kept breaking. Howard already had three implants placed and was looking at the probability of doing two more, but without addressing the bite problem, he would continue to lose more teeth and maybe even damage the implants.

Sadly, because his bite problem was not being addressed, Howard would have continued to break teeth, knock off crowns, and wear his teeth shorter over time if he'd followed the original treatment plan. Instead, he consulted me, and we decided to make models of his teeth, and took special measurements of his jaw in order to do a bite analysis. I also took a series of photos that showed the flaws that had developed in his chewing patterns. The best solution to Howard's problem involved restoring his mouth to its intended form and function. Much like restoring an older home to its optimal condition, restoring the mouth gives a qualifying patient the opportunity to experience secure chewing function and a beautiful smile, just as if there had never been damage to the teeth in the first place.

Howard chose to space his treatments over a period of four months, starting with his bottom teeth. This would establish a good foundation for the bite so that chewing forces would be balanced and smooth. When we started the upper teeth, I designed Howard's treatment plan not only so that he would look great and chew properly, but also to establish proper speech patterns and provide the right contours for healthy gums.

With the restoration of his smile complete, Howard told me that his bite had never felt better, and he's enjoying a bright, white smile without self-consciousness or reservations. He can enjoy dinners with clients or friends without worry—and he didn't have to lose any more teeth.

IT'S A MATTER OF TRUST

Howard's story was a great example of how treating only the surface problem, as he had done at first, and not addressing the root cause, which was his bite being off, did not get him where he needed to be. In his case, we discovered the root of his problem, by digging a lot deeper than typical. I pride myself on being a bit of a dental detective, and like any CSI, I have a lot of tools and technology at my disposal to track down the "perpetrator." However, in my opinion, it all starts with building a certain level of trust between the doctor and patient.

Developing that kind of trust takes time, but in my practice it starts the very first time I meet a patient. One of my mentors, Dr. L.D. Pankey, said, "I never saw a tooth walk into my office." We treat patients, not just teeth, and my first priority is to get to know my patients as individuals and give them a chance to learn a little about me. After all, the patient will eventually need to decide if the treatment they are considering is appropriate for them, if this is the right time for that treatment, and if I am the right dentist to do the work. Our first conversation is in a cozy little room, not a treatment room. Once I see that they are comfortable, I'll ask them, "How I can help you?" Some people are more to the point and tell me what their problem is right away, and other people digress, but usually within about fifteen minutes we've gotten a broad scope of what they came in for.

This preclinical conversation is very engaging, and I get a lot of necessary background before I even look into their mouths. This goes a very long way toward building trust, because people need a chance to be understood, to be treated like a person instead of a procedure. In a nutshell, my team and I strive to treat people the way we want to be treated and provide the kind of dental care that we want for ourselves and our loved ones.

EMPOWERING PATIENTS

Once we have built that trust, the next step is empowerment. I return the patients' trust in me by giving them the tools they need to be a more active participant in their dental care. As we go through each of the parts of a comprehensive exam—checking jaw joints, muscles, gums, teeth, alignment, and more—my assistant documents all of our findings so that later on, the patient and I can review them and strategize appropriate treatment. Some of that will involve a review of photographs and X-rays, but it is also hands-on and participatory. For example, if during my examination I find an area of wear or concern, during our post-exam consult, I may have the patient hold up a mirror while I point out exactly what I saw, and why it is an area of concern.

We always do oral hygiene instruction and give people information about how to massage their gums and how to access all the areas they are likely missing while brushing. If there is a problem spot, I will point it out and let them know what to do to remedy the problem, and how to monitor it properly so that it does not come back.

Sometimes I will speak to a patient about tobacco cessation, and that can be a tricky one, because most people who smoke or use chewing tobacco or "vape" are well aware of the health risks, and if they have not quit yet, either they have no desire to or have tried to quit unsuccessfully. But for many smokers, the risk of lung cancer is not something they can see; they do not think about it unless a doctor can show them a chest X-ray where something may already be developing. But I can show them exactly how tobacco causes a condition known as hyperkeratosis, a thickening of the gums, which is the body's response to the toxins in tobacco. This is something they can see and feel, and it may motivate them to quit.

Other discussions I may have with patients have to do with sleep disorders, or stress management in regard to grinding of the teeth, or breath concerns. And, of course, every patient gets the talk about diet, nutrition, and oral health.

THE DENTAL DETECTIVE

As I mentioned earlier, in some ways I fancy myself a kind of dental detective. When you come into my office with a dental problem, it is my job to deduce, "What happened here?" In many ways, I find that to be one of the most fascinating and rewarding parts of my practice.

Like any detective, I need to investigate and look for clues. If I see signs of wear such as loss of enamel, or recession of the gums, or notching of the teeth at the gum line, or cracks or mobility, then we will recommend study models. Study models are created from impressions of the teeth, and we mount them on a little machine called an articulator that's like a bite simulator. We get the models to a point where we can mimic what is going on in the patient's mouth and I can see exactly where and why their bite is off, and then we can very accurately diagnose the problem. The models will also show me if there is something simple that I may be able to do to correct the problem, and I can try it out on the models first to see if it will work and if it is safe to proceed and do the same procedure in the patient's mouth. The models will also tell me if the opposite is true and the patient will require more extensive work to correct the problem, such as fabricating a custom bite guard, seeing an orthodontist, restoring some teeth, or having teeth removed.

Beyond the articulator, I have many other tools at my disposal to do my dental detective work. Once I've gotten to know you in that initial conversation during your first visit, the next step will be to take a set of digital X-rays with our panoramic X-ray machine. This machine takes two kinds of X-rays. One is the kind that you have seen before, that shows the jaw joints and all of the jawbone, or mandible. I have found a couple of cases where there were calcifications below the jaw in the carotid artery area, and I've made referrals for the patient to go see a cardiologist. One time, the cardiologist said, "I think your dentist just saved your life." Another time, the image detected a serious bone condition that resulted from radiation treatment a decade earlier. These are examples of how these panoramic X-rays are not limited to dental diagnoses. They can also show problems with the jaw joints themselves, and show internal tumors that are out of the field of vision on a normal dental X-ray. It shows the root tips very clearly, as well as the nerve channels and sinuses. It is an amazing diagnostic tool that gives us a lot of useful information.

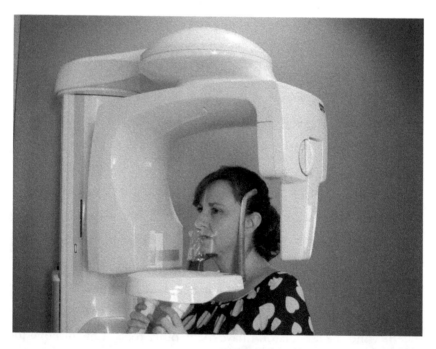

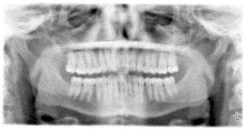
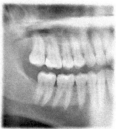
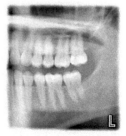

The machine also takes what are called extra-oral bitewings, which means you don't have to bite down on those tiny, uncomfortable plates in your mouth. Instead, this machine uses robotics to calibrate the patient's anatomy so that the X-rays can go between teeth and show what normal X-rays were trying to show, but without the need to put anything inside the patient's mouth.

In addition to these X-rays, we also use a lot of intra-oral photography, and the X-rays along with those photographs create a highly detailed record that we can keep going back to in order to deduce a culprit in a given case. I am still amazed at how often a patient comes in saying, "I think this tooth has moved," or "I feel a chip in my tooth that I am sure was not there before," or "My teeth look much yellower than my last visit," and my response is "Let's look at your photographs," and sure enough, the answer is right there in the documentation.

HOW CAN I HELP YOU?

All the time I spend getting to know you and getting to the root of your problems—going through the charting, showing you the imagery, reviewing your X-rays, analyzing your bite—is designed to change the patient experience. I would like patients who come to see me for the first time to walk into our office and forget everything they know, or think they know, about the practice of dentistry. I want them to know that we are going to work together to build a strategy and set priorities about what needs to be addressed and how and when we will best address it. When we look over the charts and images together, you will never see me point to something on an X-ray and give anything like a sales pitch, like "Oh, see this, that means you need four crowns and three fillings." Instead, you will hear something more like "Here's the situation, here's why it's a concern, here's what can be done about it. Your options are a, b, and c, so you let me know, how can I best help you?"

I don't know how many times a day I say that: "How can I help you?" But I say it because I don't want to do dentistry *to* people, I want to do it *for* them and *with* them.

TIPS AND TAKEAWAYS

- You are never too young or too old to start being more proactive about your oral health.

- Being too busy is never a good excuse to put off dental work. The earliest interventions lead to the best outcomes.

- Lifestyle dentistry seeks to find and address the root causes of dental issues instead of simply applying Band-Aid solutions.

- Developing a trustworthy relationship with your dental practitioner will allow you to take a more active role in your dental health.

- Advanced technology can provide a number of detailed clues to get to the root of dental problems, but it takes a dental detective who is an active listener to put all the pieces together and solve the mystery.

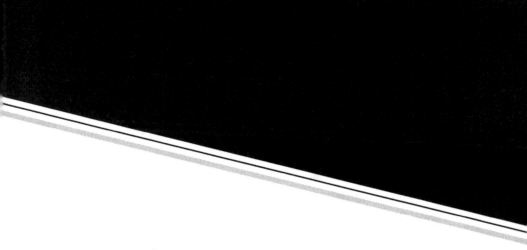

CHAPTER 4

EVERYTHING YOU NEED TO KNOW ABOUT TMD

The jaw joint is unlike any other joint in the body. While most joints hinge and some allow rotation, the jaw joint glides as well as hinges. In fact, it's the only joint in the body in which the right and left joints must work together during movement. Its name is the temporomandibular joint, or TMJ for short, and refers to the bone structures, muscles and connective tissues that together determine jaw movements. When patients experience disorders of this joint, they are said to have a temporomandibular joint disorder, or TMD. TMD can originate from imbalances within the joint itself (intra-articular) or from excessive strain of the muscles that attach to the jawbone and direct its movement (extra-articular). A healthy jaw can open wide enough to take a bite out of a fully-loaded sandwich, but where it terminates its closure depends on how the chewing surfaces of the top and bottom teeth meet.

PAM'S STORY

The tension in Pam's face when I first met her was notice-able, particularly around the eyes. She held her head rather stiffly and moved it slowly when turning side to side. She had known she had a tight and confined bite for years, but when her former dentist made a crown for a back tooth three years earlier, it never felt right and made the tooth feel sore. She kept going back to her dentist, but his response was "There's nothing wrong with the crown; the lab made it to specs," and excessive grinding on it would ruin the new crown. Over the course of three years, the problem worsened and Pam experienced shooting pain in the jaw and a slight loss of hearing. Thinking something else was causing her problems, Pam visited an ear, nose, and throat specialist, underwent a hearing test, had an MRI, and was told there was a possibility of a brain tumor causing the pain!

Pam was miserable. She couldn't chew anything on the right side for three years, even though she continued to go to her dentist's office for her six-month checkups and continued to complain about the bite problem. Each time, the dentist would refer her to another specialist.

Pam's symptoms were exceptional, but the scenario is all too common. TMD is not well understood, even by many in the medical and dental community, so the problem often goes undiagnosed or is misdiagnosed. People with TMD could be exhibiting headaches, hearing or vision problems, neck pain, or shoulder pain, sometimes for years, and think it is migraine, a sinus problem, or something else, never thinking it is a dental issue.

Bite-related problems like Pam's and the resulting TMD symptoms are often, but not always, a positional problem, not unlike imbalance problems with your hips or legs. For optimal performance, humans need balance in the body, even with jaw movements. Imagine that you have one shoe with a low heel on one foot, and one with a higher heel on the other foot. You can walk around all day, but eventually your back and leg muscles will have to take over and compensate for the imbalance. By the end of the day, you are going to be uncomfortable, possibly in pain, and definitely fatigued.

It is the same case with your jaw. Some people are very susceptible to imbalances in how the teeth touch, so if a filling or a crown is too tall or too short, it can throw off your bite, or occlusion, and that can cause the temporo-mandibular joint to be compromised. I am not faulting the dentist who originally delivered Pam's crown. The reason Pam's bite problem went undetected is that we get a limited amount of education in dental school about occlusion, how the teeth fit together, and how the jaw joint actually works. Without symptoms prior to making the crown, bite irregu-larities often go unnoticed. Personally, I was fascinated by the relationship between proper tooth alignment and TMD. I was drawn to the idea that when properly diagnosed, it can usually be easily treated, offering so much relief to people, many of whom have simply accepted chronic jaw pain as part of their lives. So, I decided to pursue advanced education on the subject and make it a specific part of my practice. Ironically, a few years after starting my endeavor to learn more about TMD, I developed symptoms myself, and there's no better teacher than firsthand experience.

The dentist that Pam had been seeing didn't recognize the problem, because he had not been trained to look for it. He thought that the lab technician had done everything properly, and that even if things may have seemed a little off, if he continued to grind on the restoration, he'd be doing more harm than good. If you just look at the teeth, that's probably true. But if he knew to look beyond the teeth to the jaw joints and muscles, he likely would have noticed that one of the joints was out of position before he even began the work. It was being held out of position by strained muscles, and those muscles were exhausted and causing pain. Think of it this way: If I ask you to hold your arm out to the side, you could do it with very little problem or effort. But if I ask you to hold it there for five or ten minutes, the muscles will start to hurt and burn, and if I then ask you to release, the arm only goes partway down, because those muscles have memory. That is similar to what happens to the jaw muscles in many TMD patients.

Once I identified the problem, we fitted Pam for a bite splint, which is a device that fits over either the upper or the lower teeth and provides balance and smoothness necessary for muscle relaxation. After a few adjustments to allow her jaw to resume its optimal position, Pam said the device was life changing, telling me that after three years in agony—and the very real fear that she had to have brain surgery—now "There's no pain. I don't have any headaches. My neck and shoulders feel good. When I put my teeth together, as long as I have my bite splint in, I feel great." Once her muscles and joints were comfortable, we were able to realign her teeth so that she also felt great without the bite splint.

Pam's case is far from unique; in fact, it is pretty typical of most of the patients I see with TMD issues. They have similar situations where they have headaches that they believe are migraines, or cluster headaches, or caused by stress, but actually, it is not any of those things; they're TMD headaches. Or, they don't know why they wake up in the morning feeling tense and exhausted. They get out of bed with their facial muscles hurting, they are tired, and their neck and shoulders are sore. What they do not understand is that what they are experiencing is a reaction to something literally being off. There is an imbalance in their body, and their muscles are overworking, trying to compensate.

While most TMD cases originate from muscle compensation issues, some evolve from direct trauma to the joints. Sometimes major trauma like automobile accidents, fistfights, or sports injuries can be to blame; sometimes minor trauma like chronic clenching or grinding from stress or sleeping uncomfortably can put excessive pressure on the joints, resulting in inflammation within the joint space. Patients with this kind of TMD may suddenly experience that their bite is off and feel tension or tenderness just in front of one or both of their ears.

Another aspect of TMD is caused by degenerative changes such as arthritic deterioration of the bone in one or both joints. These cases are more complex and require lengthier regimens of treatment, but fortunately they are rare, affecting only a small percentage of TMD cases.

PHYSICS, FORCES, AND ANATOMY

Because the TMJ can hinge, like your elbow, but also has the capability to slide right, left, and forward, it is called a "ginglymoarthrodial" joint (try pronouncing that without looking it up). Where the bones interact, they are covered with cartilage and are separated by a small, shock-absorbing disc that is there to keep the bones from rubbing together and jaw movements smooth and pain-free. Since the jawbone joins the right and left sides of the body without a juncture in the middle, balance in the right and left TM joints becomes critical.

When a patient experiences TMD pain from within the joint, it is most often due to displacement of the disc. The disc is shaped similar to a beret, tilted toward the part of the jawbone that handles the heaviest load. When we clench our teeth, or bite into something very hard, we load that area with a tremendous amount of pressure. The disc absorbs that pressure and protects the bone. If the disc is pulled out of position, it can't protect the bone, and to make matters worse, the pressure is applied to surrounding tissue that feels pain and tenderness under heavy load. Sometimes the disc slips back and forth, in and out of the heavy-load zone. When this happens, patients can often feel or hear a pop or clicking noise, though the sound is not always associated with pain.

When the teeth align properly, the healthy jaw stays centered on both discs, even with clenching. But if the teeth don't match up when the joints are in the proper position, the joints will shift to help the teeth match up; however, this may cause the joints to slip out of place. Your bite does not have to be off by much for this to occur. Think of the size of a raspberry seed. It's very tiny, but if I took a raspberry seed and glued it to one of your teeth, it would throw things off. You would notice it and play with it, trying to get it out of there so that your teeth could come to rest in a spot where the seed was no longer an annoyance. That constant fidgeting, consciously and unconsciously, when something is off in the bite is a common cause of TMD.

SIGNS AND SYMPTOMS OF TMD

The textbook symptoms of TMD include headaches (anywhere), pain and tenderness in the temple area or centered on the jaw area, back/neck/shoulder pain, or limited jaw movements. Sometimes TMD patients report an earache or a "stuffy feeling" in the ear, as if there is water trapped there. They may also experience dizziness or hear a pop, click, or "gritty" sound, like two pieces of sandpaper rubbing together, when they open and close their mouth. It's important to note that if jaw movement does not inflict pain in the jaw area, other causes of jaw pain should be considered besides TMD. It's possible for pain originating from teeth, nerves, muscles, blood vessels, and other structures to radiate to the face. Sinus problems, viral infections, salivary gland disorders, and even cancer and autoimmune diseases can all mimic TMD. The important thing is to perform diagnostic tests to get to the source of the pain, particularly if multiple conditions are overlapping and complicating the situation.

Symptoms of TMD are preceded by signs of TMD. These signs might include unusual wear on the teeth, shortening of the teeth, recession along the gum line of specific teeth, mobility of the teeth, or any kind of fractures, chips, or breaks not due to obvious trauma.

Since signs of TMD precede its symptoms, a proactive patient has the opportunity to avoid potentially painful episodes. Ignoring signs, hoping they will go away because there's no pain at the moment, is like having one foot on a banana peel; such people are taking a significant chance that they will become a victim of TMD at some point in the future.

It is for these very reasons—that patients can have signs without symptoms or symptoms without pain, or have TMD even while under a dentist's care and still not know it—that I screen all patients for TM joint problems. During a comprehensive examination, each patient gets an evaluation of joint integrity. I also have a pretty simple test that involves muscle palpation, applying two pounds of pressure—which is about what you would feel if you pressed your fingertip just to the point when your nail started to go white. I ask patients if they mind if I press on their shoulder, right on the deltoid muscle. Unless they've just strained themselves at the gym or have a shoulder injury, two pounds of pressure should not cause them any pain. On a scale of zero to ten, that would be a "zero" response; intense pain would be a "ten." Then I'll check the muscles in the neck, shoulders, and face, and then even inside the mouth, with that same amount of pressure. If I get an "ouch" or the numbers shoot up, particularly when we get around to the face, jaw, and mouth, we may have a TMD issue. Then I can get more specifically into those particular muscles where the patient felt discomfort. I divide the muscles into two groups—those that facilitate clenching—and the ones that regulate the posture or position the jaw. Identifying which muscle groups are tender and which ones are not, along with evaluating what is going on in the teeth or joint that is making the patient have a tendency to compensate, helps us both to discover the problem.

WHAT CAUSES TMD?

Many factors contribute to TMD—some of which may date back in time—which frequently overlap one another. Changes to the bite, physical injury, and clenching and grinding due to stress are common factors. Autoimmune conditions, sleep disturbances, arthritis, and discrepancies in the sizes of the upper and lower jaws can also influence dysfunction of the jaw joints.

Degeneration of the head of the jawbone, called the condyle, is the most painful and debilitating type of TMD, but fortunately it is also the rarest. Only about 2 percent of the patients I see with TMD will have this kind of joint integrity issue as the cause. I know how painful this can be, because I happen to be one of those two percenters. Before I received proper treatment, when I had a painful episode it felt like an ice pick was jabbed into one of my jaw joints. It's a very sharp, very excruciating pain, and it takes a long time to recover from it. It is also episodic, recurring periodically as adaptations inside the joint occur.

The more common cause of TMD is dislocation of the disc between the upper and lower parts of the joint. Just like a knee disc or vertebral disc, it can slip out of position, particularly if it's under strain or trauma—such as from a sports injury, but more commonly from the strain of a chronic misaligned bite.

If that's the case, as it was with Pam, we have to determine whether we can release the muscles enough to get the slipped disc back into place. This usually can be accomplished with a bite splint—a customized orthotic appliance. This approach is often referred to as "bite splint therapy." We also discuss stress management, nutrition, stretching exercises, and other supportive care. Bite splint therapy takes time, usually a minimum of three months, to get the muscles to relax and lengthen. Once that occurs, often the jaw will then realign itself, with the disc once again in its proper position, and we're back in business.

If the disc cannot realign itself, the bite splint can still work. With the splint holding things in proper alignment, nature often takes over, and the tissues behind the disc will scar over and serve as a substitute disc to cushion the two bones. In this case, you may still have the popping and clicking noise, but pain can be managed and usually avoided.

There is another category of TMD cases, where the problem is caused not by the joint but by the muscles that work the joint. If the muscles are cramping and aching, it could be because of something the patient is doing that they shouldn't be doing. We attribute a lot of these things to stress. Stress in this respect could be emotional stress that leads to tooth grinding, or it could be physical stress such as a new contour of the teeth due to a dental procedure they had. In this instance, bite splint therapy still works. The balanced contacts and smooth sliding movements of a customized orthotic device trick the brain into believing that the teeth and jaw joints are lined up. The brain then sends signals to the muscles to relax.

TREATMENTS FOR TMD

There are many ways of treating TMJ disorders, ranging from over-the-counter anti-inflammatory drugs, to custom bite splints, to orthodontics, to injections, to surgery. Left untreated, however, TMJ disorders can lead to headaches, jaw or muscle pain, and tooth damage from grinding or clenching.

If TMD has a sudden and recent onset, anti-inflammatory medications, along with a prescription for a muscle relaxer and application of moist heat to the affected area, may be all that is needed. However, chronic TMD conditions seem to recover best with bite splint therapy. A custom bite splint is a conservative approach to care and should be considered before determining whether more invasive therapies are necessary.

Of course, if the root cause that threw the bite off in the first place—such as a filling or a crown that was too high or too wide—can be corrected without further throwing things off, we will do so. Often the root cause is a slow chronic problem where maybe the teeth were filled or crowned, or maybe they were moved orthodontically, and then over time you rub hard in one particular area and finally something breaks. I often have patients who come in with a chipped tooth or broken crown tell me that it used to hurt but it doesn't anymore. That is because the break actually put their bite back into proper alignment, and they are inclined not to fix it because it resolved their TMD. But this is why, whenever possible, we try to get the bite right first, and that often involves a combination of bite splint therapy and fixing some old restorations that could have been the source of the problem.

To evaluate a patient's bite, impressions are made of the teeth, and then dental stone (similar to gypsum) is poured into the impressions and allowed to harden. The resulting models are mounted on an articulator to simulate the bite. In Pam's case, we used those models to analyze her new jaw position, and took a look at how the teeth failed to fit together properly. We could then do a preliminary adjustment to the teeth on the stone models. Using the models is so important, allowing us to know—with little room for doubt—that what we propose as a treatment can be done safely and without damaging the teeth.

Pam watched me do the preliminary adjustment with the models, and I was able to show her exactly the result she was going to get and how conservative the adjustments to her teeth were going to be. It's like having a dress rehearsal before the real event. If adjusting the models indicates that achieving balance and smoothness in the teeth will be too aggressive, other options can be pursued, like orthodontics, surgery, restorative dental work, or simply remaining dependent on the balanced bite splint.

THE BITE SPLINT

As I've mentioned several times now, the most common approach to treatment is to start with a bite splint, particularly if there are jaw symptoms, muscular symptoms, or tooth symptoms. Success rates with a custom-fit bite splint are very high in providing comfort, protecting teeth from excessive wear, and minimizing excessive load on tender jaw joints. The splint fits over either the bottom teeth or the top teeth, depending on what best fits the patient's needs. The contours on the surface of the bite splint mimic the ideal contours of the teeth, so that when the patient bites together, they feel balanced contacts on the right and left sides. Because of the balance, the muscles begin to relax, allowing the jaw joints to migrate toward the optimal position.

As the joints migrate, the bite shifts slightly, so changes have to be made in the splint periodically. When the joints have reached the ideal spot and the muscles are totally comfortable, no additional adjustments are needed. Every molar and every bicuspid is hitting just as it should, like the pistons in a well-tuned engine.

At this point of balance and comfort, we then review the patient's tooth-to-tooth relationship to figure out if they can have their teeth "equilibrated" using a conservative approach of shaping and polishing certain teeth. This can either be a negative equilibration, where you polish high spots down, or an additive procedure, where you build low spots up.

If an equilibration isn't an option, we discuss the patient's other options—orthodontics, surgery, or other restorative dental treatments. Some patients opt to simply continue using the bite splint, knowing they will be dependent on the orthotic device indefinitely, simply because they like the security and comfort of it.

WHEN TO SEEK TREATMENT FOR TMD

Just as there are a range of causes, symptoms, and treatments of TMD, the determination of when to seek help varies from patient to patient. As with any medical issue, only you can determine the impact TMD is having on your quality of life. For some folks, it's simply a noise, or a minor annoyance that they can live with; for others, it can be very incapacitating.

Most of the time, at the very least, it is uncomfortable. It can interfere with getting a good night's sleep. It limits what you are able to eat and chew. In the worst cases, I have seen people who feel completely debilitated. They don't want to get out of bed; they feel like they are hurting all over and want to withdraw from the world.

The good news is that no matter the level of TMD, we can give people an effective—and in some cases, as with Pam, a life-changing—result. And, even when we just alleviate those minor annoying symptoms such as the popping and the clicking, there's a great change that comes over the patient. You can see it in their before-and-after photos—their entire countenance seems to brighten up. Their eyes shine, their eyebrows lift. They have this buoyancy in their appearance that they didn't have before we treated the problem.

As far as when you should seek treatment for TMD, I break it down this way. Those who have a sign or two should become better educated on the condition and get to know the signs of it worsening. Those who have multiple signs should definitely be encouraged to explore treatment options. Those who have moved beyond signs, who exhibit tangible symptoms that are impacting quality of life, should be treated. And finally, those experiencing the most debilitating aspects of the disease need to know that there's hope.

TIPS AND TAKEAWAYS

- TMD is not a single disorder, but instead a collection of disorders that affect the temporomandibular joint.

- TMD is the second most common pain-causing musculoskeletal condition in the United States.

- As many as 12 percent of Americans may suffer from some type of TMD.[6,7]

---

6   "Prevalence of TMJD and Its Signs and Symptoms," National Institute of Dental and Craniofacial Research website, last reviewed July 2018, https://www.nidcr.nih.gov/research/data-statistics/facial-pain/prevalence.

7   Robert L. Gauer and Michael J. Semidey, "Diagnosis and Treatment of Temporomandibular Disorders," *American Family Physician* 91, no. 6 (March 15, 2015): 378–386. https://www.aafp.org/afp/2015/0315/p378.html.

- Women are twice as likely to be affected by TMD as men.

- In most cases, a bite splint or other noninvasive method can effectively treat TMD.

- TMD is often undiagnosed or misdiagnosed, with only one of three people with TMD seeking and obtaining treatment.

Part II

SMILE!

"A smile is a curve that sets everything straight."

—PHYLLIS DILLER

CHAPTER 5

SMILE DEVELOPMENT

There is no doubt in my mind that an embarrassing smile can hold you back in every stage of life. I have seen this time and again in the dramatic transformations we have done for children, teens, and adults that have created life-changing results. This is one of the most rewarding aspects of my career.

As human beings, we crave healthy and long-lasting relationships. We all want to be liked and accepted. Rejection can intensify feelings of depression, anxiety, and many antisocial behaviors. One basic way that we show and give acceptance to another human being is through the simple act of smiling.

For many, the link between a healthy smile and self-esteem is undeniable. This is certainly true in children. School-aged kids, and particularly teens, can be devastated by the teasing and the feelings of being a social outcast that can come with bad teeth. But it is very true in adults as well. I know both men and women who had hoped to get more out of their personal relationships, or were not as successful as they could have been in business, all because of the lack of confidence that comes with a less-than-perfect smile.

Unfortunately, I find that many patients believe that if they have a poor smile they have to accept it. They become complacent, adopting an attitude that "everybody has some kind of health issue; mine just happens to be bad teeth." Maybe they come from a family background where their parents had oral problems, and they just accept it as a given: "I am going to be stuck going through life with an unattractive smile, because mom and dad had bad teeth." Or they may have had a bad experience in another dental office, usually as a child, and they can't quite overcome their dental anxiety—leading to even more emotional difficulties on top of the self-esteem issues and the anxiety they already have with regard to their poor smile.

If there is one message I want the reader of this book to come away with, it is that it doesn't have to be that way. There are things we all can do, especially as parents, to ensure that we, and our children, develop and maintain a healthy smile for life.

STARTING OUT RIGHT

We all want our children to start out in life on the right foot, but it's just as important that they start out on the right tooth! What parent isn't elated by their baby's first smile, or when they see those first tiny two front teeth come in? Parents need to take that joy and pride a step further and look at it from their child's perspective over the course of growing up, and realize how important it is for them, as parents, to do everything they can to protect and preserve that precious smile.

When a child has a healthy, bright smile, he or she gains social acceptance and can build confidence and overall good self-esteem. When a child comes to see me and he or she has problems with his or her teeth, whether they're crooked or overlapped or decayed, I see a shadow cross over that child's face. Often, children with inferior smiles feel like they are not as socially accepted as those with good teeth. It can be a huge blow to their self-esteem. Parents need to be proactive early on. I gave my own children fluoride when they were very young. Did you know that the American Pediatric Association has said that tooth decay is the most common chronic disease in children in the United States, and recommends the use of fluoridated toothpaste at six months of age or upon tooth eruption? I agree with the APA's recommendation. Children do not even have very many teeth at six months, but the teeth are developing under the gums and the fluoride gets in the bloodstream and makes the teeth harder before they erupt into the mouth. There has been a lot of controversy about fluoride, but in the recommended amounts, it has proven to be very beneficial in fighting decay.[8]

Basically, the time to start proper care of your teeth is as soon as they come in. Those first teeth can come in anytime, typically from one month to one year, but no matter when they arrive, it is up to parents to take care of them until the child is old enough to do so for his or her self, just as they do for every other aspect of their baby's health.

Parents need to understand that children's teeth are not the same as adult teeth, and that they need some special care. Also, if your child's teeth do become decayed or damaged, we do not have as many options to repair them as we do with adult teeth, because of these differences. Children's teeth do not have the same level of mineralization

---

8   U.S. Department of Health and Human Services Federal Panel on Community Water Fluoridation, "U.S. Public Health Service Recommendation for Fluoride Concentration in Drinking Water for the Prevention of Dental Caries," *Public Health Rep* 130, no. 4 (Jul–Aug 2015): 318–331, https://doi.org/10.1177/003335491513000408.

as adult teeth, which means they are more susceptible to damage and decay and are also that much harder to repair. The bonding materials that we use in dentistry work better on adult teeth than they do on children's teeth.[9] We will still use bonding and similar materials to make repairs, but it will not make as tight a seal or last as long as the repair would on an adult tooth. This is because the material simply does not adhere to them as well, due to the lack of mineralization. This is all the more reason why I want to emphasize how important it is to really protect those first teeth.

While bonding materials may not adhere as well to children's teeth as they do to adult teeth, something that does adhere well—and which I highly recommend from a preventive standpoint—are dental sealants. Dental sealants are a specific type of resin that's bonded to the deep grooves on the chewing surfaces of your teeth. To the naked eye, the grooves look like a shallow V-shaped groove, but when you look at them under a microscope, you can see how deep they really are. Debris can easily get in there, and bacteria follow. The bacteria produce acids as their waste products, which causes tooth decay. This is why most of the time that kids get cavities, it is on the chewing surfaces of the teeth, where these grooves are. In fact, the majority of decay in kids occurs on the biting surfaces.

When the teeth first erupt, we can scrub those teeth really well, clear out those grooves completely, and then apply this resin, the sealant, so that it penetrates into the tooth structure, effectively sealing the groove so that food and debris cannot get in there anymore. It can significantly cut down on decay. Sealants can be applied to baby teeth, and then again as they are replaced with permanent teeth.

---

9   Deniz C. Can-Karabulut et al., "Adhesion to Primary and Permanent Dentin and a Simple Model Approach," *European Journal of Dentistry* 3, no. 1 (2009): 32–41. https://www.ncbi.nlm.nih.gov/pmc/articles/PMC2647957/#__ffn_sectitle.

There is one thing I need to point out about sealants, and I do have to tell this to parents and even adults who get them for the first time. Just because you've had a sealant applied does not mean that you now have some impenetrable force field on your teeth and can go out and eat as much candy as you want and not follow other good oral habits. Sealants are a great proactive method, and they can reduce your risk of getting cavities by about 60 percent, but they cannot and do not prevent all decay.

BABY TEETH ARE NOT DISPOSABLE

A problem I often run into in trying to get parents to take a more proactive role in their child's smile development is an attitude that you do not have to pay that much attention to baby teeth, because they are going to fall out anyway. Nothing could be further from the truth. Baby teeth are not disposable. The truth is, you really do not want to lose your baby teeth prematurely, because the baby tooth acts as a kind of guide, like a jungle guide clearing a path through the brush with a machete, for the permanent tooth to erupt in the proper position. It also serves to hold the position for the permanent tooth, keeping adjacent teeth from drifting or tipping into the space. If that tooth is removed prematurely, then the eruption of the permanent tooth may be off. This can lead to crowded, misdirected teeth and all sorts of orthodontic problems.

So, baby teeth play a vital role. Besides the obvious benefits of smile, speech, and nutrition, you want your child to retain their baby teeth so that they lose them when they should, which then allows for adult teeth to come in as they should. This pattern helps establish an ideal jaw position as the new teeth grow into their proper functioning position. Premature loss of baby teeth can upset this natural cycle. And, of course, taking baby teeth seriously, and training your kids how to respect them and take care of them properly, sets your kids up for a lifetime of good dental habits and good oral health.

BRUSHING UP ON HOW TO BRUSH

"Brush your teeth!" We have all heard our parents say it. But do you recall them ever telling you any more than that? They may have told you when to brush, but did they ever really take the time to tell you *how* to brush? Most parents probably have not, and it is not their fault, because they probably were never taught proper brushing and flossing techniques themselves. One of my goals is to break that cycle, by teaching adults everything they need to know about brushing right so that they can pass that on to their kids. The question I am asked by parents most often is "What is the right age to start my kids brushing on their own?" When to start depends on the development of the child, but as a rule of thumb, at two to three years of age, you can make brushing into a game, where you and your child take turns brushing one another's teeth.

Take a soft-bristled child's toothbrush and use it to gently massage the child's gums. This way, you impart the feel of the brush on the gums and get the child to understand that they must scrub at the gum line as well as the teeth. Then, let the child hold your toothbrush and gently rub your teeth before trying it on themselves. This gives them a feeling of how many teeth there are and how far back they go, so that they can brush without poking themselves in the throat, or gagging, and making brushing an unpleasant experience. As they are brushing your teeth, show them how they have to go inside and outside, up and down. As they start to brush on their own, it's important to make it a game, make it fun, and be sure to reward them when they do it right. (But please do not reward them with candy. I had one parent who gave her kid M&Ms for brushing at night!) Using a progressive chart—where they earn a sticker each time they brush right and a certain number of stickers adds up to a toy or a fun experience—is a good way to go.

Other things that are important when teaching your kids to brush right from an early age are:

- Be sure to use the right size of toothbrush. You want something small that can fit in the smaller nooks and crannies of the baby teeth.

- Use a child's toothpaste, because most adult toothpastes are too strong for children.

- A fluoride mouth rinse is good to use, such as ACT anti-cavity treatment. These can be found in most grocery or drug stores.

Brushing correctly has to become part of the morning and night routine. I know that nighttime is tough. Bedtime can be the worst time of day for parents, because they're exhausted, and they just want to get the kids off to bed. Make brushing part of the nighttime routine, but maybe not right before bed. Have your kids brush, say, before they are allowed a half-hour of TV or before they can read for a half-hour before going to bed, so that it is part of the nighttime ritual but not necessarily the last thing they do before going to sleep. This will make it a little easier on you and will make your kids less likely to associate brushing with bedtime, which could make them less inclined to brush.

THE ROLE OF ORTHODONTIA AND EARLY INTERVENTION

I am not an orthodontist, and when I see patients—kids and adults alike—who are in need of orthodontia, I refer them to an orthodontist. However, I would be remiss in my duty as a dental professional if I did not discuss the value of early orthodontic checkups and early orthodontic intervention. Most parents do not realize how early they can have their kids screened for orthodontic issues, believing they have to wait until all of the child's permanent teeth are in. However, the orthodontists I work with recommend doing a screening of children between the ages of five and seven, to see if their growth and development is on target for a correct bite. Screening early can detect problems early, and may result in less aggressive straightening procedures. In fact, I know this from personal experience. I have two sons and two stepdaughters, who were eight, nine, ten, and eleven, respectively, at the time of our marriage. All four kids ended up having orthodontic treatment, but for one of my daughters, the treatment would have gone faster and easier if she had received treatment at an earlier age.

Usually, when orthodontic problems are detected early, they can be treated in ways that do not require a lot of dental hardware. For example, if the lip muscle on the bottom lip is very strong and very tight, it could be forcing the growth of the teeth toward the tongue rather than more vertically or canted out toward the lip. In this case, we can use a retainer called a lip bumper, and when the kids wear it, it basically gives the teeth a fighting chance against that strong muscle, allowing the arch to elongate. That is only one of the many examples of where we can do some minimal work on a kid's teeth and possibly avoid the need for a more complex treatment when all of their permanent teeth come in. A lot of parents make the mistake of waiting until their kids are twelve or thirteen years old to have them screened, and many times that could be too late to influence growth patterns.

Another misconception that people have about orthodontic work is that it is only for kids or teens. Today, many adults are wearing braces for the first time, especially since we now have aesthetic options such as tooth-colored brackets, clear orthodontic trays, and even braces that are applied to the inner surfaces of the teeth. There are also cases where adults have to have braces for a second time, after wearing them as kids, perhaps because they did not wear their retainers as long as they should have after their braces were removed, or they slipped back into other bad habits that may have caused their teeth to shift in the first place. I treated one lady who did not finish her last time in braces until she was seventy-two!

TOOTH TRAUMA

Besides tooth decay and misalignment, if there is one more very important thing that parents need to be aware of and try to avoid during early smile development, it is tooth trauma. Kids will fall; it is part of growing up. Often those incidents will lead to tooth trauma. There are two things to know about tooth trauma. One is that when it can be avoided, it should be, so when your kids are involved in competitive team sports, encourage them to wear proper mouth gear. The second is that if a tooth is broken or knocked out, it is vitally important that it gets the proper treatment right away. Often, improperly treated childhood tooth trauma results in dental problems later in life.

This was the case with Jerry.

JERRY'S STORY

High school sports, particularly boys' football, have high injury rates. Jerry's accident had occurred decades earlier when he was on the practice field and, without his helmet, he jumped into a "dog pile" and cracked his head against someone who was wearing the appropriate protective equipment—and knocked out a front tooth. Jerry's parents immediately took him to the dentist, but their finances were scarce and the options to replace his missing tooth were limited in those days. The dentist made a mold, and from that, a retainer-type device with a replacement for the missing front tooth was fabricated. The device was removable, which was annoying, and it wobbled when he chewed. Also, it was made out of acrylic, which didn't hold up well over time.

Several years passed, and Jerry decided it was time to take the next step and have a cemented replacement made. However, cosmetic dentistry had not developed to where it is today; his bridge was made of gold, with tooth-colored acrylic across the front. His smile was uneven as well, because as a young adult he had lost back teeth and had not had the opportunity to replace them. The adjacent teeth drifted into the spaces, and the opposing teeth hyper-erupted into the available space. Over time, the

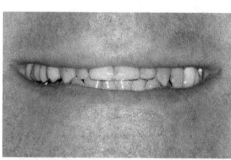
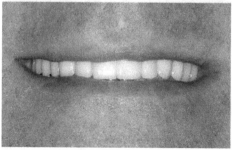

tooth-colored acrylic darkened and Jerry subconsciously limited his smile.

When we began his dental rehabilitation, Jerry had considerable anxiety about undergoing treatment. His experiences with dental trauma and disappointing results from earlier in life haunted him. Even so, he mustered the courage and determination to correct the dental problems that had plagued him most of his life. After multiple visits over the course of a few months, his missing teeth were replaced, his bite was back to normal, and he had a naturally beautiful smile. By the way, Jerry is my brother.

FIRST AID FOR TOOTH INJURIES

Parents need to know what to do if a child falls and damages a tooth. Every time a tooth is injured, even if it appears to be a minor chip, it should be examined by your dentist. It's good to take an X-ray at the time of the trauma and then look again, say, six weeks down the road. We may be able to tell the parent in advance that the tooth may darken, but also tell them not to panic—darkening is better than losing the tooth at this point. That is always the goal with a tooth injury in children—to try to save the tooth. Even if your child's tooth is knocked out, there's a chance it can be saved. When a tooth is lost:

- Handle the tooth very carefully. Try not to touch the root of the tooth.

- Clean the tooth by rinsing it, preferably with milk. If milk is not available, rinse it with water.

- Try to reinsert the tooth into the socket and have your child bite it into place.

- If you can't put it back, keep the tooth moist, drop it into a glass of milk if possible, and transport it that way to your dentist's office as soon as possible.

Here is a basic first aid kit for dental emergencies that every parent should have on hand:

ITEM	PURPOSE
Gauze	Bleeding
Orajel	Toothache
Advil	Swelling
Clove oil (applied with small cotton pellet)	Deep cavity
Tweezers	Applying cotton pellet
Frozen peas (used as an ice pack)	Swelling, pain
Soft picks or floss	Removing food debris
Orthodontic wax	Covering sharp edges
Milk	Rinsing an avulsed tooth
Vaseline	Temporarily replacing crowns or temporaries
Salt	Warm saltwater rinses for irritated gum tissue
Disposable gloves	Helping someone with a dental problem
Dentist contact info	Calling your dentist as soon as possible

TIPS AND TAKEAWAYS

TOOTH DEVELOPMENT BY AGE AND STAGE

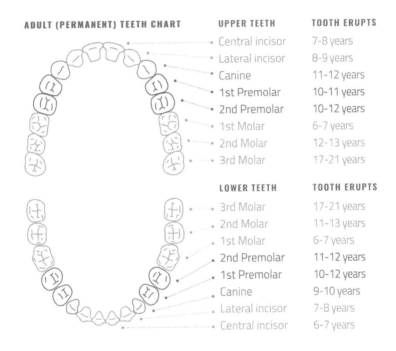

ADULT (PERMANENT) TEETH CHART	UPPER TEETH	TOOTH ERUPTS
	Central incisor	7-8 years
	Lateral incisor	8-9 years
	Canine	11-12 years
	1st Premolar	10-11 years
	2nd Premolar	10-12 years
	1st Molar	6-7 years
	2nd Molar	12-13 years
	3rd Molar	17-21 years
	LOWER TEETH	**TOOTH ERUPTS**
	3rd Molar	17-21 years
	2nd Molar	11-13 years
	1st Molar	6-7 years
	2nd Premolar	11-12 years
	1st Premolar	10-12 years
	Canine	9-10 years
	Lateral incisor	7-8 years
	Central incisor	6-7 years

What Parents Need to Be Aware of at Each Stage:

- Primary teeth are forming during pregnancy; good nutrition is of great importance for the development of those teeth.

- Guidelines for tooth eruption are just guidelines. Some children fall outside of the average age ranges.

- Teething can make your baby irritable or fussy and may cause drooling and loss of appetite.

- Check labels on teething rings and don't buy one with phthalates or bisphenol A (BPA) listed in the ingredients. Also, don't buy one with liquid inside, as the child might perforate the ring and ingest the fluid.

- Buy a teething ring made of firm rubber (check the label) and refrigerate it so the coolness can soothe the gums.

- Toddlers who are getting their back molars may feel relief from a low-sugar popsicle.

- Some children grind their teeth in their sleep. While this is not uncommon, it is best to have a dentist evaluate the child for sleep problems or loss of enamel.

- Your child should be checked by an orthodontist by age seven. This allows time for preemptive treatment.

- Studies indicate that fluoride, in proper doses, has beneficial effects on dental development and prevention of cavities.

- Whether or not your child should have fluoride supplements to reduce the chance of decay depends on many factors; ask your dentist what is most appropriate for your child.

CHAPTER 6

STUNNING SMILES

Did you know that researchers have found that a beautiful smile not only makes you more attractive, but also makes you seem more intelligent, interesting, successful and wealthy to others? According to a study conducted by the American Academy of Cosmetic Dentistry in 2004:[10]

- Virtually all Americans (99.7 percent) believe a smile is an important social asset.

- Ninety-six percent of adults believe an attractive smile makes a person more appealing to members of the opposite sex.

- Three-quarters (74 percent) of adults feel that an unattractive smile can hurt a person's chances for career success.

10   Anne E. Beall, "Can a New Smile Make You Look More Intelligent and Successful?" *Dental Clinics* 51, no. 2 (April 2007): 289–97, https://doi.org/10.1016/j.cden.2007.02.002.

The good news is, modern dentistry has the means to help just about anyone obtain a beautiful, radiant smile.

I did not win the genetic lottery when it comes to beautiful smiles. As a child, my teeth were crooked and asymmetric, and some teeth were pointed. Early on, this wasn't a problem, but by the time I was in middle school I started noticing how my mouth looked different than everyone else's, and I became more self-conscious about my smile. I started to smile less and put my hand over my mouth more. In high school, I was very embarrassed by my smile. Even styling my hair, putting on makeup, or dressing stylishly didn't erase my feelings of inadequacy regarding my unattractive smile. To this day, I still feel a twinge of embarrassment when I look at my high school pictures. Even in my prom pictures, when everyone else is smiling I'm wearing a tight-lipped grin.

I have seen firsthand how being embarrassed about a smile can inhibit people. You become shy and withdrawn, leading others to think that you're less outgoing or less friendly. They may even think you are arrogant or self-absorbed, when actually, you have just withdrawn because of your discomfort over your smile.

A SMILE MAKEOVER

The good news is that, thanks to the many options we have in cosmetic dentistry today, no one—child, teen, or adult—needs to go around with an embarrassing smile. From orthodontics and whitening, to implants and veneers, we have the tools to give a person a complete smile makeover. I have found that when people get the smile they've always wanted, it lights up their face and puts a noticeable sparkle in their eyes. It's almost as if they've had a face-lift—without the surgery! I don't mean to diminish the efforts that estheticians and plastic surgeons can have on fine lines and unwanted wrinkles, but what will catch a person's eye across the proverbial crowded room is a confident smile and sparkling eyes.

When you see some of the cases that we have on file, it's really jaw dropping to see how we could take ten years off this women's face, or how we changed this man's persona and gave him back the confidence he needed to succeed in the workplace. In order to help our patients who are considering a smile makeover to visualize the probable results, I will often Photoshop a photo of them smiling, correcting their smile for unevenness, discolorations, and asymmetry. If they like the photos, the next step is to verify the same corrections on stone models of their teeth. One lady requested our Photoshop version of her smile for her profile picture on Facebook! I guess she couldn't wait for the real results.

Sometimes a smile makeover is as simple as smoothing rough edges and sending the patient home with a whitening kit. Other times it can require veneers, crowns, orthodontic work, or a combination of various techniques.

Veneers

Veneers are a very common cosmetic dental technique, and they can make a world of difference. Veneers are ideal to restore chipped, cracked, discolored or misshapen teeth. We can even use them to close spaces between teeth to some degree. Veneers are a thin layer of porcelain (or sometimes composite resin) and are custom made to fit over teeth, providing a very natural and attractive smile. I find that there is a lot of misconception about veneers. Some patients are concerned when I mention them, because somehow, they have this mental image that we have to grind down their teeth excessively to affix the veneers. We do have to shape the tooth to a degree before putting on a veneer, but it is such a tiny degree, usually less than a millimeter. A millimeter is equivalent to the thickness of a credit card. Basically, we are only taking off a very thin layer of enamel to replace it with the veneer.

DONNA'S STORY

Donna had watched enough episodes of television makeover shows to know that a brand-new smile was available with porcelain veneers. She even did some research on how much a makeover would cost, since dental insurance doesn't typically cover these elective procedures. When we first met, she knew what she wanted and told me how much she expected it to cost, but her estimate was about 20 percent too high. When she realized the true cost was lower than she anticipated, she couldn't wait to begin the work. After closing unattractive spaces and changing the color from a rather dark shade to white, she looked radiant; in fact, she looked several years younger. She later told me, "Getting porcelain veneers is, by far, the best gift I have ever given myself."

Donna's results with veneers are very typical. When done correctly and properly cared for, veneers can last ten to fifteen years. I have had patients who have gone more than twenty years without needing their veneers replaced. The key to successful veneers, as it is with so many other dental procedures, is to make sure we address any underlying bite problems first, such as making sure the gums are healthy and there are no issues with the bite being off. If we do that before we affix the veneers, they look great and last a long time.

Crowns

Sometimes a smile makeover requires crowns, or what people more commonly refer to as a cap. Whereas a veneer is a thin overlay on the front surface of the tooth, a crown is a little thicker and completely encircles the tooth. A crown is indicated if there is significant damage to the inside surface of the tooth, if we need to change the inner contours of the tooth to enhance the chewing function, or if the tooth would be stronger by being completely restored. Like veneers, crowns can be used to make teeth look straighter or to close spaces. When I say the word "crown" to some patients, they get a mental image of old-fashioned porcelain-to-metal crowns with a dark area at the gum line. For many years now, we have eliminated that dark line, as well as the unnatural opaque look of those outdated crowns, with all-ceramic crowns that transmit light like real teeth and blend seamlessly into the natural tooth.

TRISTAN'S STORY

Like most teenagers, Tristan had a rebellious streak. He resented being told what to do, and that included following instructions while he was going through orthodontics. He refused to brush, much less floss, to the point that the orthodontist felt the braces should come off before the teeth were damaged from all the debris around the brackets. Once the braces were removed prematurely, not only were Tristan's teeth still crooked, but he also couldn't chew well because they didn't connect, or "occlude," well either.

Tristan's parents tried to reason with him, get him engaged in the situation and take responsibility for his part of the solution. When he said fine, he'd do better next time, they found another orthodontist to straighten Tristan's teeth. The braces were placed, but again Tristan refused to brush his teeth, and this orthodontist also aborted the process for fear of excessive decay.

Tristan was in his early twenties by the time his parents brought him to me to see what, if anything, could be done to improve his smile. He now wore a baseball cap with the brim pulled down low over his brow. He never smiled and seldom spoke. Whenever he did speak, he mumbled and did not make good eye contact.

When I examined his mouth, I found that not only were the teeth crooked and didn't occlude well, he had rampant decay and his gum tissues were red and swollen. It was time for a frank discussion, but this time Tristan was no longer a minor, and the conversation did not involve the parents; this was just between the two of us. I told him my story, how as a teenager I was told I'd lose all of my teeth by the time I was forty, and how debilitating I felt that would be. I told him he was living the same story, that he—and only he—had a choice to make, and very little time to make it before it would be too late to have any options to save his teeth. I told him flat out, that even if he made the choice to try to save his teeth, it would take a lot of effort, not just in the beginning of treatment, but for the rest of his life. In fact, I told him, I wouldn't even agree to start treatment until he proved he could maintain it. The first step was to teach him how to clean his teeth. He was to return to my office in two weeks to show me what he could accomplish.

When Tristan returned for a checkup, I could tell that he was actually trying to change his behavior. I praised his efforts, made some suggestions on how he could do an even better job, and rescheduled him for another checkup appointment. To make a long story short, over the next few months, Tristan began to collaborate in the process of not only saving his teeth, but restoring them to full health, function, and beauty. With Tristan's newfound commitment and his parents' generosity in providing their son with the needed dental care, the design process began. Because he had cavities in so many areas, he needed to have crowns; veneers were not an option.

As we made over his teeth into a beautiful smile, a transformation took place in Tristan's self-esteem as well. The baseball cap disappeared. He made eye contact when he spoke. In fact, at one point, Tristan came to my office and as he was being escorted to a treatment room at the end of the hallway, he stopped to talk to other patients he encountered. He truly blossomed, and before long he told us he had a girlfriend. I followed Tristan's case for several years before he moved away, and he always stayed on track with excellent home care for his second chance at a beautiful smile.

In the completed makeover, crowns and veneers can be indistinguishable. In fact, in many patients, their new smile can be a combination of both crowns and veneers, and sometimes the crowns are on natural teeth and sometimes they are on implant replacements.

DENTISTRY BY DESIGN

Donna's and Tristan's cases are good examples of what we mean by "Dentistry by Design." In their cases, as in all our smile makeover cases, we literally design a new smile from the ground up. This means that whenever we do a cosmetic case, we don't just schedule the patient and put them in the chair and start working. When I see a cosmetic case in the very beginning, it's very exciting because I can already see in my mind's eye what the outcome is going to be. But to get there, we will start with photography. We often move things around in Photoshop to see what would be required to give the right smile line or gum contours—we consider the shape, the spaces, the texture, things like that. Then we have models made and design the patient's smile on the models first, which could involve several hours of work. We make sure that the bite is correct on those models, then we add length, or shorten things, or rotate them, all by using dental wax. From that wax design, we can get a balanced, aesthetic look that we can make a template out of, and from that template we have a predictable outcome that we can share with the patient. We can work with the models to give the patient exactly the look and comfort they want. Some people like curved, and some people like corners, and once we get that design just right and the patient is happy, it's a simple process to communicate those guidelines to the lab technician.

Working with qualified lab technicians is something that distinguishes exquisite dental practices from the rest. These technicians are true artists, and their skills and services deserve recognition, because they are an integral part of the team that is working to give patients the excellent results they desire.

LOOKS GOOD—FEELS GOOD—LASTS A LONG TIME

The ultimate goal of any cosmetic dental procedure is for me to provide my patient with something that looks good, feels good, and will last a long time. I find it a little bit funny that over the years, we have developed this subspecialty known as cosmetic dentistry, when actually all dentistry is cosmetic dentistry in a sense. Even if I am doing something that is purely functional or therapeutic, such as filling a cavity, ultimately I am not simply removing the decay and repairing the tooth. When I am done, the filling should look aesthetically pleasing and as close to your own natural tooth as possible.

Conversely, all cosmetic dental work should start with the patient's oral health in mind. I have seen cosmetic dental work that looked good on the surface but was not healthy where it counted. It didn't respect the gum tissues, or it didn't take into account proper occlusion. I have had to repair failures because of those kinds of issues with older dental work. It's a global situation, so you have to look at the whole mouth. You could treat just the bite, but then you wouldn't have a cosmetic resolution. You could treat just the cosmetics, but then you would leave dangerous components in place that may damage the work you've just provided. It all has to work together. You need healthy joints and healthy supporting tissues and good function overall, as well as a pretty smile. The final part of the equation is that the patient has to keep up their end of the bargain, by adopting good oral habits and doing their due diligence at home. When this all comes together, you wind up with a smile that looks good, feels good, and will last.

TIPS AND TAKEAWAYS

- Veneers are a thin layer of porcelain or composite resin custom made to fit over teeth, providing a very natural and attractive smile.

- Direct Resin Veneers are applied directly to the teeth and can be completed in one visit, usually without the need for anesthetic.

- A crown or cap is a prosthetic device that is cemented or bonded to a broken or damaged tooth.

- Once in place, crowns and veneers can be indistinguishable.

- Veneers are used to improve the outer surface of teeth; a crown is needed when the other surfaces are involved.

- Cosmetic procedures work best, and last the longest, when any underlying bite issues are resolved first.

CHAPTER 7

A LIFETIME OF SMILES

A healthy smile is important throughout life, yet it impacts each stage of life differently. A baby's first smile is one of his or her earliest forms of communication; a toddler's smile indicates joy and happiness; for teens, smiles are so important for self-esteem and first crushes; for adults, a smile may be the first step toward personal relationships or career advancement; and as we enter our senior years, maintaining a healthy smile could be key to being able to still eat what we love and to enjoy quality of life.

"ALL I WANT FOR CHRISTMAS IS MY TWO FRONT TEETH..."

When it comes to kids, of course tooth decay, sweets, and brushing is an issue. But still, one of the greatest threats to kids' teeth is accidents. For instance, there was the time I received an emergency call from a frantic mother on Christmas Day. Remember the movie *A Christmas Story*, where the only thing the boy Ralphie wants for Christmas is a Red Ryder BB Gun, and everyone from his parents to Santa tells him "you'll shoot your eye out, kid"? This particular mom had a son about Ralphie's age, his name was Blake, and he'd received a BB gun that morning as a Christmas gift. He didn't shoot his eye out, but he aimed the gun at a flat rock on the ground and the pellet ricocheted back and hit his two front teeth.

I immediately met Blake and his parents at my office to assess the damage. There was a good-sized triangle of space where the two front teeth normally touch—thank goodness that pellet didn't hit his eye! It was a fairly simple procedure to repair the damage with tooth-colored bonding material, which not only gave him back his smile, but also protected the exposed tooth surfaces from pain and sensitivity to cold air, foods, and liquids. He looked like himself again and would be able to chew normally, not to mention he'd be spared the teasing that he'd inevitably have to face from his friends, especially if he had to explain he had shot out his own teeth!

Some years later, when he was in his early twenties, the bonding was starting to show signs of discoloration and wear, as that material was inclined to do. Together, with his parent's approval, we decided to convert the case to porcelain veneers. We knew that Blake was still growing, and that we'd have to redo the veneers again in the future. However, at the time, it was important to give him an attractive smile during those awkward teen years and into his young adult years.

Blake is now about thirty-five years old and drives over three and a half hours from where he currently lives to see me for his dental work. We've agreed it's time to redo the veneers to account for changes due to his growth, and this time the veneers will most likely last even longer. The fact that he drives so far to see me is heartwarming. It shows an appreciation, not only for the quality of my work, but an even deeper appreciation for the fact that someone cared about protecting him from embarrassment and discomfort, and still does.

A TEEN'S TALE

Young kids can be very cruel, and that is why it was so important to me that we restored Blake's smile for him when we did. But sometimes, I think to myself: Blake was a rough-and-tumble boy, and if we couldn't do what we did, physical issues notwithstanding, maybe socially he could still have gotten through adolescence with two broken teeth. Biting into an apple would have been problematic, but maybe other boys would actually have found the way he got them knocked out funny, or he could have made up some story about how he lost them in a fight, and he still would have made friends and all.

Not so much with girls. If there is any patient I see who is dealing with more self-esteem issues related to a poor smile, it's a teenaged girl. Acceptance and peer pressure is a daily part of a teen girl's life. Unlike boys of that age, teen girls who feel self-conscious about their smile get it from both sides. They compare themselves to the popular pretty girls and also may feel they could never get the cute guys to notice them. Middle school and high school can be especially difficult for a girl with a compromised smile.

KATE'S STORY

Baby teeth are supposed to have spaces between them, so when you see gaps in a five-year-old's smile, it's cute. But when you're a teenager and you have spaces between your teeth, it can be a problem. That was the case for Kate, a beautiful sixteen-year-old who had just gotten out of braces. Now, wait a minute—I know what you are thinking.

Aren't braces supposed to close those gaps? Not necessarily. Kate's orthodontist realized that in order to provide her with proper chewing function and a long-lasting result, it all depended on the proper positioning of the roots of her teeth, even if that meant there would be gaps between the teeth when the orthodontic work was complete. The finalization of the case would require cosmetic treatment, and that's where I came into the process.

Kate came to my office about a week before her braces were due to come off. We made impressions of her teeth and measurements of her jaw joint so that the models could be mounted on an articulator to simulate her bite and chewing function. The stone models were adjusted so that wax could be added to the undersized teeth to give them adult-sized contours. On the models, everything looked proportionate and the chewing motions functioned well, so a template of the proposed tooth contours was created. This would serve as a 3-D template to guide the procedures so that we could achieve the same results in Kate's mouth.

The big day came just one day after Kate's braces were removed. The template from the lab design allowed me to follow the predicted outline using a glass and resin composite material that bonds directly to the tooth. First a layer of translucent material was used, then a layer of tooth-colored composite, then tints and enamel-like finishes. Within a few hours and without any anesthetic, Kate's smile was transformed from a childlike, gap-toothed smile to the smile of a lovely young woman.

When Kate first saw her new smile, she laughed, and then she said what I was hoping to hear: "I love it!" Then she hugged me—twice. Moments like those are why I love my job.

ADULT ANECDOTES

As we move away from teenaged angst of peer pressure, acceptance, and first dates and enter young adulthood, an attractive smile
continues to have an impact on our physical, emotional, and now, as
an adult, even our financial well-being. I have known many a patient
who feels he or she did poorly on a job interview, or was passed
over for a promotion, because of a less-than-perfect smile. Indeed, in
many ways an attractive smile is part of the American Dream.

DIANE'S STORY

"I want an American smile," Diane stated flatly, as if there
could be no confusion on my part as to what that meant.
"Tell me more," I urged her.

Diane was born in the United Kingdom and grew up
at a time and in a culture that didn't have easy access to
orthodontics, whitening, or other cosmetic dental options.
By the time she moved to the United States, she observed
that many people in America had straight, white teeth, and
she decided that getting a beautiful smile was something
she needed to attain to fit in and look "more American."
In addition to wanting a more American smile, she also
decided to get in better shape, and committed to a new
diet and fitness regimen. Diane's children were in their
early teens at this point, and she felt the time was right to
take some steps toward self-improvement after years of
nurturing others.

Diane's teeth were a bit uneven and somewhat square
looking. A few were slightly rotated. While some of the teeth
were a bit dark, others were a medium shade. As usual, we
began with a thorough exam and made models of her teeth

that could be altered to give the desired cosmetic result. I determined that porcelain veneers could give her the look and feel of her so-called American smile while conserving the most natural tooth structure. Since Diane's broad smile revealed almost all of her top teeth, we would revamp her smile from molar to molar.

When selecting a shade for veneers, I generally recommend considering complexion and eye color, especially the "whites" of the eyes. If the teeth are quite a bit whiter than the whites of the eyes, the teeth tend to stand out too much. On a comical note, while we were discussing Diane's color choice for her new veneers, I told her that with her blond hair, blue eyes, and dark tan, she could go quite white and it would look natural on her. To that, Diane replied, "Well, I'm not really a blond, and I'm wearing blue contact lenses. For that matter, my tan is a 'fake bake.'" We laughed, but she still chose a bright white shade and, to use one of her favorite words, it looked "fabulous" on her.

Diane was a trooper. In spite of the long preparation appointment, she later told me that the procedure seemed quite easy and she would recommend it to anyone who wanted to improve their smile. When I asked Diane if she was happy with the results, she said, "I am thrilled and delighted!"

Meanwhile, she was diligently working toward her health and fitness goals. She became leaner and stronger and eventually became certified as a personal fitness trainer. But she didn't stop there—a few years later she established a workout facility that became so successful that she had to buy additional land for expansion. Did having her teeth restored factor into her later success? I imagine her success was the result of hard work, long hours, and a ton of determination, but it didn't seem to hurt her achievements to have an "American smile."

Can a better smile help advance your career and success? Diane's story is just one of many where I saw that to be the case. I cannot say whether or not in those cases it was because they looked better to their employers or customers, or because of the way their improved smiles increased their own confidence and self-esteem, but the fact of the matter is, beautiful, straight white teeth and a winning smile are among the first things we notice when we meet people, and we make an instant judgment based on that smile. That can possibly advance a career, and it certainly factors into matters of the heart.

ALEX'S STORY

Alex was a very shy young man. I had known and treated him as a kid, but his parents divorced, and I am not really sure what happened, but I did not see him for a number of years. He came back to see me when he was in his twenties, and he had what we call a reverse smile. His front teeth were a little shorter than his eye teeth and his back teeth, so when his lips went up, his teeth went down. I could tell this really affected him; he seemed even shyer and more introverted than he was as a child.

There was a problem with fixing Alex's reverse smile: When he bit together, the edges of his bottom front teeth were already hitting the chipped edges of his upper front teeth. If his lower jaw was in its proper position, this was going to require a couple of years of braces before we could move forward on the cosmetic corrections.

During the diagnostic evaluation, I determined that Alex was posturing his jaw forward, forcing those front teeth to hit with excessive force. In fact, it was actually the way his back teeth touched that encouraged this to happen. By aligning the teeth to the proper, and more relaxed, jaw position, we gained all the room we needed to correct his smile.

How do I know? A few years after we completed his restoration, he connected with me on Facebook and asked me to come to his wedding, because he wanted "the lady who fixed his smile" to celebrate in the fact that he had met someone and was going to marry her. And that made me very happy!

SENIOR SMILES

The so-called golden years can be very tarnished for a senior with tooth problems. Everybody knows how important it is to plan for your retirement from a financial standpoint, but many people fail to plan to keep their smile, and do not realize how important that can be. Suppose you've envisioned yourself sailing around the world, climbing mountains, traipsing through Europe experiencing the wonders of French cuisine and the splendors of Italian wines or Belgian chocolates. Dental problems, and particularly missing teeth, can literally take a bite out of any such retirement plans.

Tooth loss, of course, can impact your ability to chew, taste, and enjoy food, but did you know that studies indicate tooth loss can take as much as ten years off your life?[11]

---

11   P.K. Friedman and I.B. Lamster, "Tooth Loss as a Predictor of Shortened Longevity: Exploring the Hypothesis," *Periodontology 2000* 72, no. 1 (October 2016): 142–52, https://doi.org/10.1111/prd.12128; "A Recent Review Article Posits That Tooth Loss May Predict Shortened Longevity," ADA website, Feb. 3, 2017, https://www.ada.org/en/science-research/science-in-the-news/a-recent-

When people are young, I think they shrug off how important teeth are to enjoying happy and fulfilling senior years. Too often, they think, "So what, I will just get a denture." People who do not wear dentures have no idea what an inadequate substitute for your own natural teeth they are. Just as a prosthetic arm or leg that replaces a lost limb, the denture that replaces missing teeth is an inferior substitute for the real thing. For most denture wearers, foods taste blander, and the perceived temperature of food is diminished. While a few denture wearers adapt well to a mouth full of acrylic, most have trouble chewing hard or crunchy foods and regret the loss of their natural teeth.

If you went to your doctor, and he told you that you had a condition that meant you have to eat a soft diet for twenty-four hours, you would probably say, "Okay, I could have scrambled eggs and mashed potatoes for a day." But if he said, "I want you to have a soft diet for the next three months," that would probably be a lot harder and not so enjoyable. Now imagine if your physician said, "You can have only soft foods for the rest of your life." That would be devastating, wouldn't it?

Now for those who have dentures and want something better, there is hope. Implant-supported teeth can eliminate the bulk and instability of dentures, but surgery is required, and as of this writing, a fully restored mouth costs a minimum of $50,000 in most areas of the United States. That is what people who are not planning for future dental health could be facing, and most people don't think this through and realize how important it is to be more proactive

review-article-posits-that-tooth-loss-may-predict-shortened-longevity; David W. Brown, "Complete Edentulism Prior to the Age of 65 Years Is Associated with All-Cause Mortality," *Journal of Public Health Dentistry* 69, no. 4 (Fall 2009), 260–2, https://doi.org/10.1111/j.1752-7325.2009.00132.x.

about their teeth and gums. I tell them it's like having an IRA for your mouth!

TIPS AND TAKEAWAYS

- A healthy smile is important in every stage of life.
- You are never too young or too old to be proactive about dental care.
- The link between a healthy smile and self-esteem is evident at every stage of life, with different impacts.
- Tooth loss can shorten lives.
- Dentures are a poor substitute for natural teeth in later years and can severely impact your quality of life.
- If you buy your kid a BB gun, make sure they know not to fire at flat rocks!

Part III

LIVE!

"Take care of your body. It's the only place you have to live."

—JIM ROHN

CHAPTER 8

THE MOUTH IS THE GATEWAY TO GOOD HEALTH

It has been said that the eyes are the windows to the soul. If that is true, then the mouth is the foyer to the health of the body!

It may not always be as simple as healthy mouth, healthy body—however, if things are not healthy in your mouth, most likely you will also be experiencing problems in other areas, because inflammation, which is the root of most disease states, doesn't stay isolated to one area of the body. For example, if you have diabetes and it expresses itself as an infection in the foot, that infection is not limited to the foot; it will eventually spread throughout your body, wreaking all sorts of havoc. Most folks seem to understand that intuitively with regard to the rest of their body, but for some reason they neglect or overlook the mouth/body connection, and fail to realize that the same thing that can happen in a foot or a finger can and does happen in the mouth—with gum disease, tooth infections, or just general poor oral hygiene.

It is also a two-way street, in that if you have systemic problems in the body, they also affect the mouth.

YOUR DENTIST AS YOUR FIRST LINE OF DEFENSE

Since the mouth is kind of a gatekeeper to your body's health, in a very real sense, your dentist could be your first line of defense. There needs to be a change in the perception of dentists—from simply the people who fill cavities, to true medical professionals responsible for your overall health and well-being, working in collaboration with your primary care physician—and we are seeing this start to happen.

CLAY'S STORY

I just had a patient, Clay, come in a week or two ago, and during my usual examination, I noticed that the inside surfaces—the lingual surfaces—of his teeth were eroded. I realized we needed to discuss gastroesophageal reflux disease, or GERD. Clay said, "Oh yeah, I had that, but that was a long time ago." We were considering doing quite a bit of work on his teeth, and I didn't want to take any chances of the work being destroyed if he still had an issue with acid reflux, so I urged him to see his gastroenterologist.

To make a long story short, a few weeks later, Clay made a special trip back up to my office to thank me, because the gastroenterologist did an endoscopy and found that Clay had Barrett's esophagus, which is precancerous. They told him they'd discovered it early enough, but that he would have to be on a prescription medication for the rest of his life to minimize the possibility that the condition would advance to esophageal cancer. Now, thanks to this intervention, the chances of him ever developing cancer in his esophagus are slim to none.

But had he not listened to me and not gone to see the gastroenterologist, the outcome would have been very different. So he thanked me "for essentially saving my life," when really all I did was notice the telltale signs that were right there in his teeth that perhaps other medical professionals had missed. Many MDs have confided in me that they do not spend a lot of time in medical school on oral health. During a routine physical, most physicians are taking a tongue blade and looking down your throat, but they're not really observing the teeth, and they're not looking under the tongue and under the neck unless there are specific symptoms to lead them there that the patient may be complaining about, such as "I've got a pain here." But usually by the time it hurts, it's too late, especially in the case of a lesion or something that could be oral cancer.

LINDA'S STORY

Several years ago there was a lady, let's call her Linda, who came to see me with a painful lump under her tongue. When I looked at it, I was astounded to see a large, ulcerated growth that looked very painful indeed. She told me, "Well, I've had it for eight years, but back then they did a biopsy and it came back fine." I explained to her how tests sometimes have false negatives and false positives. "Let's get you to a throat specialist," I said, "and take a closer look." A new biopsy still came back negative, but this time they also did an MRI, and they found that there was cancer at the core of this tumor, deeper than the biopsy had sampled. The only lifesaving treatment was to surgically remove the affected half of her tongue. As horrible as that sounds, it could have been much worse. She's alive and she's functioning well to this day, thanks to that second series of tests.

Sometimes, because of the different diagnostic tools we have available to us, dentists can routinely see things that other practitioners would have to go out of their way to discover. For example, panoramic X-rays can reveal quite a bit about what may be lying beyond the teeth and the gums. Impacted wisdom teeth, cysts, tumors, calcifications, and even foreign objects can pop up on panoramic images. I remember getting a call from a patient on Thanksgiving Day, but the call was about the patient's mother, who was visiting from out of town. She had inadvertently bitten down on a turkey bone and chipped a tooth. Because she was feeling quite a bit of pain, I arranged to meet both of them at my office. Normally, I would have taken an X-ray of just the tooth in question, but something in the back of my mind kept prodding me to take the more revealing panoramic X-ray. I've learned to listen to this inner voice, or intuition, so I took the broader X-ray. Immediately, I could see a worrisome anomaly in the back of the jawbone. I fixed the chipped tooth, but I told her that when she got home she really needed to see her doctor about what I had seen on the X-ray. It turns out she'd been treated for breast cancer years before, and the cancer had returned and had metastasized to the jawbone by way of the lymph nodes.

We as dentists are on the front lines and have the skills and abilities to catch many health issues, and not only oral cancer. There are indicators in the mouth of things such as GERD, as in Clay's case, as well as diabetes, heart disease, sleep apnea, and a number of other conditions. You have to stop looking only at a patient's teeth and start looking at the whole person.

HEALTHY HABITS FOR A HAPPY MOUTH

If keeping our mouths healthy can be a key to overall health, what kind of things should we do, and not do, to keep our mouths as healthy as possible? Basically, if you think about it, you already know. Think about the typical laundry list your doctor would recite. "Well, these are the things you need to do to stay healthy and live longer. Eat a good diet, don't smoke, consume alcohol in moderation, get enough sleep, etc." Those are basically all the right habits for your mouth as well, and it all works in conjunction. If you live a healthy lifestyle for your body, it will work for your mouth, and vice versa.

However, beyond the kinds of foods to eat and those to avoid that I mentioned in early chapters, and the coaching on brushing and flossing, there are some specific healthy habits for better oral health.

Besides a diet heavy in sugar and processed foods, smoking and tobacco use is probably one of the unhealthiest habits there is for your teeth, mouth, and gums. I understand how difficult smoking cessation can be. And I see many patients who've made the difficult decision to quit smoking because they realize the risk of lung cancer but then switch over to chewing to get their tobacco fix, not realizing the risk of oral cancer from chewing tobacco is many times greater.

I've read that when you smoke, there are over seven thousand different toxic chemicals in the smoke that you are exposing your mouth and lungs to.[12] One of the effects of those chemicals on the mouth is that they cause capillaries to shrink, which reduces blood

---

12   "Tobacco," National Biomonitoring Program, Centers for Disease Control and Prevention, last updated April 7, 2017, https://www.cdc.gov/biomonitoring/tobacco.html.

flow to the tissues. When that occurs, you are much more prone to gum disease. Restricted circulation also means you're a slower healer, which can get in the way of doing some needed dental procedures, such as extractions, or implants if you lose teeth due to gum disease from smoking.

But then if you switch over to chewing tobacco to get your fix, you are exposing your mouth to those toxins even more, literally bathing your teeth and gums in them. The link between smokeless tobacco and oral cancer has been well documented, and smokeless tobacco increases your risk of other cancers as well. Studies have shown that those who chew or dip tobacco are also at an increased risk of esophageal cancer and pancreatic cancer. And yet, the tobacco companies continue to position smokeless tobacco products as a safe alternative to cigarettes.

I understand that a lot of people like to have a drink every now and then, and most of us realize the systemic problems alcohol abuse can cause, but few realize just how damaging excessive drinking can be to your dental health. According to the Oral Cancer Foundation, "Although tobacco use has been proven to increase the risk of oral cancer, people who use both alcohol and tobacco are at an especially high risk of contracting the disease. Scientists now believe that these substances synergistically interact, increasing each other's harmful effects."[13] It seems that the alcohol dehydrates the cell walls of oral tissues, which makes it easier for the tobacco carcinogens to penetrate. In addition, heavy drinking is associated with nutritional deficiencies, which can lower the body's ability to use antioxidants to fight cancer.

Illicit drug use is another thing that dentists can detect. In particular, cocaine and methamphetamine cause a reduction in saliva

---

13 "The Alcohol Connection," The Oral Cancer Foundation,
   https://oralcancerfoundation.org/understanding/alcohol-connection.

flow that results in a characteristic pattern of decay, affecting the entire mouth. It should go without saying that for a healthy mouth, not to mention a healthy mind and body, stay away from unlawful drugs.

But it's not just recreational drug use. You might be surprised at the number of over-the-counter medications and prescription drugs that can have a negative impact on your oral health. A side effect of many medications is dry mouth, and dry mouth can lead to a number of dental issues. Not only do we need saliva to moisten and cleanse our mouths and start the digestion of food, but salivation also prevents infections and gum disease, by helping to curtail bacterial and fungal growth in the mouth. Dry mouth is a common side effect of many prescription and nonprescription drugs, including drugs used to treat depression, anxiety, pain, allergies, and colds. So if you are taking such medications, it is a good idea to use an oral rinse, such as Biotene, to restore mouth moisture.

A RECAP OF WARNING SIGNS

If you think of your mouth as the guard at the front gate, trying to keep your body healthy, what then are the alarms that should go off letting you know you have a problem? First and foremost, particularly when it comes to oral cancer, never ignore a lump, bump, pimple, or lesion in the mouth that lasts for any significant length of time. There are any number of sores and such that can occur in the mouth; most are minor and are treatable or will resolve on their own. However, anything that lasts more than two weeks, gets larger, changes shape, or causes pain should be looked at by your dental professional immediately. But if you wait to the point of pain, that can often be too late. It is always better to be safe than sorry. Don't forget the case of Linda: don't ignore a lesion in the mouth because it doesn't hurt or because you can live with the pain. Sometimes people know something may be wrong but don't want to see the dentist, because they're afraid of what the outcome will be. But one of the simplest things we can do is take a tiny little brush and scrub that spot lightly, pick up some cells, and send them to a lab—and know for sure.

The early warning signs of cancer are not the only warning signs you need to be on the lookout for. There are many warning signs of gum disease you should be aware of, such as:

- Red, swollen, or tender gums or other pain in your mouth

- Bleeding while brushing, flossing, or eating hard food

- Gums that are receding or pulling away from the teeth, causing the teeth to look longer than before

- Loose or separating teeth

- Pus between your gums and teeth

- Sores in your mouth

- Persistent bad breath

Any of the above can be a sign of serious infections that can lead to tooth loss. Signs of other dental issues could include the popping and clicking typical of TMD, pain, tooth sensitivity to cold or hot, or dry mouth.

TIPS AND TAKEAWAYS

THE DOS AND DON'TS OF GOOD ORAL HEALTH

	DO	DON'T
GENERAL	• See a dentist for regular checkups. • Brush twice a day using a soft-bristled brush. • Floss once a day. • Brush your gums and the back of your tongue as well as your teeth. • Follow your doctor's recommendations for periodic X-rays.	
FOODS AND BEVERAGES	• Drink plenty of water. • Eat whole, unprocessed foods.	• Drink sugary sodas or sports beverages. • Eat frequent sweets, particularly those with prolonged exposure. • Eat excessive amounts of chips, crackers, pasta, or other refined foods.
TRAUMA	• Wear a mouth guard for contact or high-intensity sports.	• Use your teeth to open containers or bite into non-food items.
BLEEDING GUMS	• Manage red, swollen, bleeding gums with regular dental cleaning, visits, and consistent daily home care.	• Ignore persistent bleeding of the gums when flossing. • Ignore chronic bad breath.
CAVITIES	• Tell your dentist about areas sensitive to hot or cold temperatures, or sweet foods.	• Wait until you feel pain to get it checked. • Depend on antibiotics for relief of tooth pain.

BITE DISEASE	• Protect your teeth with a night guard or retainer if you are aware of nighttime clenching and/or grinding. • Consider orthodontic braces or restorative dentistry to correct chronic bite problems.	• Disregard popping and clicking of the jaw joints. • Overlook wear or breakage of the teeth.
COSMETIC CONCERNS	• Explore possible treatments to obtain a beautiful smile.	• Assume you can't afford cosmetic dentistry.
ORAL CANCER	• Have any lesion that lasts more than two weeks checked by your dentist.	• Assume a "negative" biopsy result is 100 percent accurate. • Use tobacco products or drink excessive amounts of alcoholic beverages.
SYSTEMIC HEALTH	• Be alert to a dental connection to sleep disorders and the resulting health problems associated with them. • Be aware of the damage to teeth from GERD and other bite problems. • Know that heart disease (and other health concerns) are directly related to gum disease.	• Ignore warning signs. • Ignore you dentist's advice to see another medical practitioner.

CHAPTER 9

AN OUNCE OF PREVENTION

The great baseball player Mickey Mantle once said, "If I had known I was going to live this long, I'd have taken better care of myself!" The "Mick" may have been known to have a bit of a sense of humor, but his sentiments are essentially true. However long you may have to live, life is too short not to enjoy every minute of it. And, taking care of yourself—for life—includes taking care of your smile. There really is no need to go through any stage of life—particularly your latter years—with missing or damaged teeth, because once you know the warning signs, so many oral health issues are largely preventable.

I cannot stress enough how being proactive about your teeth, mouth, and gums is so much healthier in the long run. It is not only better for your overall health and outcomes, but in most cases it's also a lot less expensive to treat problems early than to deal with further complications later on. Think about it this way: if you hear a little rattle in your car, you know you'd better get to the mechanic right away and fix it when it may just be a hose—rather than let it go until suddenly you have to replace the engine!

It is the same with dental care, and yet I still find that most people are *reactive* when it comes to a mouth or jaw problem rather than *proactive*, and that is usually based on pain. We react to pain as indicative of a problem, but in most dental concerns there are plenty of warning signs of an issue before you feel pain, and by the time you do feel pain, you are usually at the most advanced stages of the problem, requiring the most expensive and extensive interventions.

This is particularly true in the case of gum disease. If you wait to address gum disease until it hurts, you are at the very least looking at a long and protracted battle to try to save as many of your natural teeth as possible, and more than likely looking at dentures or some other full mouth restoration, such as full arch implants. Whereas, if you understood and heeded the early warning signs, such as puffy or bleeding gums, we could have intervened sooner, and most likely prevented any tooth loss. Similarly, in TMJ patients, if you come in when it does not hurt but you hear the characteristic popping and clicking or you notice wear or chipping on the teeth—instead of waiting until you have pain in your jaw—we probably can correct the problem with a bite guard rather than more extensive therapies, or even surgery.

FRANK'S STORY

I had this one patient, Frank. He had been very reactive when it came to his oral health, taking what I call a one-tooth approach. He would have a problem, get it fixed, and not see a dentist again until he had another problem. Then he would get that problem fixed, and so on and so on.

Unlike most patients, Frank had a pretty good reason for taking this approach. As a commercial airline pilot, Frank felt that he simply did not have a lot of time for complicated dental work.

I met Frank when he broke one of his front teeth and had to have it removed. He was now sixty-five, and he was missing nine permanent teeth. He was losing both his smile and his ability to chew. Being a pilot, Frank had a mechanical mind, and he quickly grasped the concept of the functional role that teeth play in chewing. He began to understand now how one-tooth dentistry had facilitated the decline of his teeth over time.

We had to look at his case from a global perspective—to not only repair the damage but also protect his remaining teeth. Using models to plan and design the optimal outcome, we created a strategy that would achieve his goals and yet stay in his budget. Worn teeth had to be restored, even though they had no decay. His bite had to be balanced so that new restorations fit a mechanical chewing scheme. As we executed the plan, his smile blossomed into a handsome grin that suited him perfectly. Frank changed in his expression and engagement with me and with the others in the office. It was as if a light came on inside him, and it glimmered in his eyes.

Frank was now very pleased with his smile, but had he been more proactive in the beginning, he probably wouldn't have lost the teeth he'd lost, he wouldn't have the chipping and breaking, and he would have saved himself a whole lot of time and money.

Someone once said that when it comes to your health, you are going to have to pay one way or another. There is a price to pay for education, and a price to pay for lack of education. The latter is almost always more expensive than the former. What you choose to spend your money on is largely up to you. This is beautifully illustrated in a poem that appeared in Dave Grant's *The Great Lover's Manifesto*.

There is a price to pay for education.
There is a price to pay for ignorance.
There is a price to pay for attending to good health.
There is a price to pay for neglecting health.
There is a price to pay for attending to relationships.
There is a price to pay for neglecting relationships.
There is a price to pay for love.
There is a price to pay for fear and hate.
We cannot choose whether we pay—
only for what!
—Dave Grant, *The Great Lover's Manifesto*

BEING PROACTIVE: WHAT TO LOOK FOR

As mentioned, education really is the key to being more proactive about dental health. People really cannot be blamed for ignoring the signs if they do not know what to look for.

One reason that people may wait too long to take care of a problem is that as adults, our teeth are somewhat less sensitive than they were when we were kids. For most of us, the nerves in younger teeth react much more quickly to sensations such as hot, cold, or sweet than the nerves in older teeth. This is because the nerve chamber in young teeth is quite large, but over time the nerve chamber becomes more calcified and tooth sensation is diminished, sometimes even obliterated. If adults wait for that pain signal they felt in a small cavity as a child, they may very well need a root canal or extraction by the time they feel it in their mature tooth. So waiting for pain, or some other sensation such as being sensitive to hot, cold, sweet, or sour, as an indicator of a dental problem is not as effective in an adult as it was when you were a kid.

So, if we cannot rely on our sensations so much, what kinds of things should we be looking for before something hurts? As I mentioned earlier in the book, "Signs precede symptoms." Here are some signs you can watch out for:

- It seems you keep experiencing broken teeth, loose crowns, or missing fillings.

- Your teeth look short or worn, and they're prone to chipping.

- Your teeth have developed a very flat smile line.

- You notice gum recession, but only in certain areas.

- You seem to get food trapped in the same places with every meal or snack.

In 1977, businessman Burt Lance popularized the phrase "If it ain't broke, don't fix it," and many people take the same attitude with their dental issues. I actually keep an elegant Waterford water glass in my office for times when this quote comes up. I'll set the valuable etched glass on the table and say, "This glass 'ain't broke,' so it doesn't need fixing, right?" Inevitably, the patient agrees. Then I move the glass closer and closer to the edge of the table, until part of the base is hanging over the edge and the patient is showing some concern. "This is your condition," I'll say. "It's not broken, at least not yet, but each time I've seen you over the last couple of years, it's getting closer and closer to the edge. If you wait for it to break, it may shatter into a thousand pieces and may be impossible to fix." Doesn't it make more sense to intervene when we detect the signs of disease rather than wait for its symptoms?

Even though kids are more sensitive to indicators of potential dental problems, it is still very important that parents get to learn and recognize the early warning signs of a problem in their kids, because a child may be afraid or embarrassed, or lack the ability to see or articulate a problem before they are in pain, and by then it could be too late to prevent a more serious issue. One thing parents can do is to inspect their children's mouth, and if they see something like dark spots on the teeth that don't go away with brushing, that's definitely a warning sign of underlying decay. Of course, it is incumbent on parents to be conscious of good nutrition, and to limit sugar as we have said. I realize how difficult that can be for some parents. If you are struggling with a kid with a chronic sweet tooth, I ask you to look back at the chapters where we mentioned healthier alternatives to sugary snacks. But if you try your best and you know for a fact that your kid is eating more sweets than they should, then you need to be even more aware that they may be prone to decay, and be even more proactive about looking for the warning signs, teaching good brushing and flossing skills, and getting your kid on a pretty consistent six-month regimen so that they are examined regularly for decay. I also urge all parents, and particularly those of kids who they think may be predisposed to decay, to consider dental sealants and fluoride treatments. Sealants can be applied to baby teeth, and then again as they are replaced with permanent teeth, really cutting down on decay. I know that some parents wish to avoid fluoride for fear of toxicity, but when used by a dental professional, in the right amounts, it is very safe. If I did not think so, believe me, I never would have given it to my own children when they were quite young.

Crowding can be another big issue with children. If your baby teeth don't have enough space between them, that's a red flag, because we want to see little bitty teeth in spaces that will be big enough when the full-sized teeth come in to replace them. If your kid has tightly packed teeth, that is all the more reason not only to get them to the dentist on a routine basis to monitor the level of the crowding, but also to take them to an orthodontist earlier than you would imagine. Most parents think, "Okay, when my kid is twelve or thirteen, we'll go to the orthodontist." In a crowding situation, there's actually a growth and development problem, which indicates that they should be screened at about age seven. In fact, I know several orthodontists who recommend first screenings at about age seven even for kids who are not exhibiting crowding.

BEING PROACTIVE: BEING ABLE TO SEE MORE

Knowing what to look for at home certainly helps my patients be more proactive about their dental health. But that is only part of the picture. I also have many more tools at my disposal today, which can help me see more. Panoramic X-rays, for example, can see deeper and reveal more about oral problems at far earlier stages of development, as long as you are a diligent dental detective and know what to look for.

For example, I had this one patient, a woman in her sixties, who came in to see me. Since she had not been to a dentist in a while, as part of her workup we did a panoramic X-ray. The scan revealed that she had a cyst that had formed around an impacted wisdom tooth that had never been properly addressed. She knew there'd been a wisdom tooth left behind many years before, but nobody had ever felt it needed to be taken out, because it was basically inert and seemingly not causing her any pain or other problems. So it just sat there for decades, until I happened to take a panoramic X-ray as a part of her routine screening and found the cyst growing around that impacted wisdom tooth. These kinds of cysts are not uncommon, and they are almost always benign, but they can lead to complications if left untreated. This one definitely needed to be removed. I referred her to an oral surgeon, and as it turned out it was about the size of a robin's egg when the surgeon removed it. He said that although benign, it had grown inside the jawbone for so long and was so large that it had gotten to the point where it had made the periphery of the jawbone so thin that all it would have taken was a minor bump to shatter her jaw like an eggshell. She was walking around with the proverbial glass jaw and had no idea!

EARLY INTERVENTIONS LEAD TO THE BEST OUTCOMES

The case I mentioned at the head of this chapter, about the airline pilot who could have done so much better if only we'd seen him sooner, is a very common scenario. People have so many reasons for not going to the dentist, but the most common ones are time and money—which is kind of ironic, because I have found that, almost always, if you put off a problem, you are only going to wind up costing yourself more of both. If you wait longer than you should, thinking you're going to save money by not coming in to see your dentist, in the long run you are going to spend more money, and most likely are going to need more time off from work or from enjoying your leisure activities, because we are going to need more visits for more complex restorations.

TIPS AND TAKEAWAYS

- Do not wait until you feel pain as the indicator of a problem. By the time any given dental condition is causing pain, it may already be too late for a simple fix.

- Learn to recognize the early warning signs of dental problems.

- In children, look for dark spots on the teeth that do not go away with brushing.

- Look carefully at your smile each day in the mirror. Get to know it well. Do not ignore it if something seems "off." It is not normal for teeth to wear, chip, or break over time.

- Look for crowding of teeth in children.

- Look for the early warning signs of gum disease: red, swollen, or puffy gums, and/or pain or bleeding when brushing.

- Do not ignore any growth or sore in the mouth that lasts more than two weeks, changes, grows larger, bleeds, or causes pain.

- Smoking and excessive consumption of alcohol increase your risk of developing oral cancer.

- New technologies such as panoramic X-rays allow dentists to see more kinds of problems, at earlier stages.

- Try not to make excuses not to see your dentist. Early interventions lead to the best outcomes.

CHAPTER 10

TAKING CHARGE— BE PROACTIVE!

We have arrived at the last chapter of this book, and by now I hope you have come to realize not only the value of being proactive about dental health, but also that much of the power to do so is in your hands. It really all comes down to choices. You can choose to eat the right foods, you can choose to become better educated about home dental care, you can choose not to ignore warning signs, and so and so on. Making the choice to **Eat** (right), **Smile** (more often), and **Live** (happier and healthier)—is largely up to you!

IT'S NOT JUST TEETH

When it comes to a lifetime of smiles, we are not only talking about your teeth and how they look. We're talking about function—the supporting tissues, the teeth, the jaw, the smile—and beyond that the mouth-body systemic connection. Function mostly has to do with the jaw, the joints, and the muscles—their movement and interactions. To be proactive in that regard, you need to not make the mistake that so many people do and ignore the popping, clicking noises that are a warning sign that things may worsen in the future.

If you hear that kind of noise, even if there is no pain, have it checked. If you have jaw problems, if your bite is off, we need to correct that first. If you do need more extensive dental work, if we fix the jaw issues first, then those restorations will have better and longer-lasting outcomes. So, identifying problems early—and fixing them in the proper order—is just another way of being more proactive about your dental health.

As far as most issues related to function, you really need to listen to your body. If it's giving you little hints and clues that something is not right, then it's so much easier to get you back on track early in the process than to wait for everything to derail and then try to get back on track.

When I am talking about being proactive about the supporting tissue, think about the "pink stuff." There are your gums, your tongue, your throat, and your cheeks, as well as what you do not see, the underlying bone. The bone itself can give you very few clues, but it is bone loss that most often leads to tooth loss. With bone loss, a lot of times you don't have any pain, but the teeth are losing their support, and people are shocked when they lose a tooth that never hurt, never had a cavity or showed any signs of decay. But the fact is, the foundation was being eroded underneath. It's like having termites in your house and not knowing it, until one day you step right though the floorboards!

But bone loss is the result of gum disease, and so if you can pay attention to the signs of gum disease—bleeding when you brush or floss, redness, and swelling—then you can take care of that before the bone disappears and the foundation gives out!

Furthermore, when it comes to your gums, as we mentioned in earlier chapters, if there is an infection or inflammation around the teeth at the gum line, then there's a very good chance that there is infection and inflammation throughout the body. That does not mean taking proper care of your gums can guarantee that you will never have heart disease, or some other problem with systemic inflammation, but it can promote better overall health, and lower your risk for other diseases.

YOU ARE NEVER TOO YOUNG OR TOO OLD TO BE PROACTIVE ABOUT DENTAL HEALTH

While being proactive about smiles for life is not only about teeth, that doesn't mean you should ignore the many stories your teeth can tell. You probably know your own reflection better than anybody. If you look at your smile and your teeth don't look right, they're probably not right. If they're worn and canted and short, then it's an indication of poor function. And again, the sooner you intervene, the easier the remedy, and the less expensive it is, too. A lot of people see a chip or a crack, and they think that it happened because of a single event, such as when they bit too hard into a nut or something. But in reality, often that chipping and cracking is a perpetual problem that has been caused over time by a bite issue.

You can also see signs of decay long before a cavity hurts. But even if they see darkening or holes, in the absence of pain many people mistakenly think it is not something they have to worry about until it hurts. But again, the longer you wait, the more it is going to cost you in time and money. There is not a single dental issue that you can point to—from a simple cavity to a major infection—that is not going to get worse as time goes on and require more extensive treatment the longer you wait. Just ask Gerry.

GERRY'S STORY

Gerry was an engineer with an oil company in Houston, but he was assigned to an oil refinery project in South America. For decades, he flew back and forth between Texas and Venezuela, spending most of his time at remote locations along the Venezuelan coast. That meant it was easy for him to rationalize that he didn't have time for dental visits. The truth was, he was terrified of being in the dental chair.

Many years passed and upon retirement from his occupation, he returned to the states full time. He couldn't rationalize his avoidance of dentistry anymore, and he drummed up the courage to see me. There aren't many things I haven't seen in my thirty-plus years of practicing dentistry, but I'd never seen a case quite like Gerry's. His years of neglect had led to multiple cavities, severe gum disease, and orthodontic problems that coalesced into a tremendous challenge, even for a restorative dentist like me. Of course, I was determined to save every tooth that I possibly could, but I had to bring up the probability that Gerry was going to need dentures, with or without implant support underneath.

But Gerry surprised me; he was willing to do anything and everything to save as many teeth as possible. He had the funds to do the work, and with retirement, he had the time. He also had a stubborn tenacity to make amends for previous poor decisions and a determination to overcome his fears.

So we went to work with a treatment plan. He would need to lose some hopeless teeth and see a periodontist to immediately manage his gum disease. He would need to see me for decay removal between his other appointments, and he would need to consult an orthodontist to make some challenging corrections to his bite. In the midst of his braces, implants would be placed so that they could heal in time to use them as anchors for the final stages of braces. And finally, I would restore his mouth with crowns and veneers to complete the process. I called a meeting with the two specialists and coordinated a strategic plan. Gerry was all on board.

It took a few years to complete Gerry's case. He became an ideal dental patient—never missed an appointment and became engaged in the entire process. He followed the advice given to him and dutifully maintained his dental health with good home care, a nutritious eating plan, and routine dental visits. By the end of his protracted treatment, he had never been healthier, both dentally and medically. As for his fears, they pretty much disappeared. When I would leave him in the operatory to go into my lab for a few minutes, he'd follow me, just to continue our conversation, and he'd casually watch me work as I trimmed and polished his temporary crowns.

You could say that Gerry should have become proactive about his dental health earlier in life, and I would agree—that would have saved him having to go through much of the dental treatment he underwent. But he is also my poster child for the idea that you are never too young, or too old, to be proactive. The fact that he became proactive, even in his mid-sixties, created a turn of events that ensured his overall health and well-being for the remainder of his life.

There is a lot of scientific evidence that Gerry's risk of heart disease, diabetes, arthritis, dementia, and even cancer diminished significantly when he became more proactive about his dental health.[14]

14   J. Kim and S. Amar, "Periodontal disease and systemic conditions: a bidirectional relationship," *Odontology / the Society of Nippon Dental University* 94, no. 1 (2006): 10–21, https://doi.org/10.1007/s10266-006-0060-6.

The truth is, it is never too early, or too late, to think about dental care—even at the end of life, as our next story illustrates.

JIM'S STORY

Jim was a prime example of a patient being very proactive about dental health, and he always made time for regular cleanings and other routine visits. In fact, he was a really fun patient, who liked to drive a sports car and take the curves on the windy roads. He was full of life and humor. We got along really well and I liked him a lot. We'd only known each other for a couple of years when I found out from his wife, who was also a patient, that he had become ill and that he was staying at home due to the illness.

Then one day I got a phone call from him and a note to please call him back, and when I did he informed me that he had been in the hospital for quite some time and was now restricted to bed. He had a hospice nurse attending to him and he was housebound, in the final stages of a terminal disease. He was not going to be leaving the house at all anymore, and he and his family had made the decision that he would die at home. He contacted me because on top of all that he was facing, a tooth had started bothering him, and he was having this ache and wanted to know if there was anything I could do about it. Knowing he was living on borrowed time, he hoped to spend his last hours with his family in the comfort of his own home, not dealing with a toothache.

I talked to his hospice nurse and prescribed the correct medication to relieve the pain, but I also reassured Jim that I would make a house call if necessary. Not that I would really need to, but just to let him know that he had that ace in the hole and that if we needed to take a tooth out to make him comfortable, we'd certainly do that. I remember saying, "I may have to use a flashlight. It might be ugly, but we'll get it done." He laughed and he thanked me so much.

Some time later, his wife came back in for a visit. She told me that Jim had passed away, peaceful at home, as he wished. She also told me that the hospice nurse, having been impressed with my efforts to ensure Jim's comfort and my willingness to make a house call, had asked her, "Where did you find this dentist?" The wife smiled and said, "I can give you her name." So I was pleased with that. I felt like I gave him some comfort there at the end. Jim's story is literally illustrative of taking charge of your dental health from cradle to grave.

I WON'T GO TO THE DENTIST BECAUSE...

Jim may have been a good patient who came in for regular checkups and dealt with problems as soon as they arose, but when it comes to reasons—or more accurately, excuses—as to why someone refuses to see their dentist, believe me, I have heard just about every one of them.

As we have mentioned before, cost or perceived cost is often a prohibitive factor. But, once again, I have to emphasize, if you let something slide, it is only going to go from a simple treatment to one that will be more expensive in the long run. People think, "Well, I'll just wait until I have to have it pulled." But even if you stop at simply having the tooth pulled—which is never really recommended—that extraction alone is going to cost a lot more than had you had the cavity filled way back when.

But if you decide to replace the tooth with a prosthetic, the median cost of a dental implant in the United States at this time is around $5,000 per tooth. If you take the value of thirty-two teeth times five thousand dollars, suddenly you have a new perspective of the value of a healthy mouth! But, even if things have deteriorated and you have a lot of work to be done, we can always develop a treatment plan that allows payments over time, or there may be a health credit line, or we may be able to do the work in phases so that you only pay for one part of the project at a time. Every dentist I know is willing to work with patients to deliver the necessary treatment and stay within the patient's budget, or else refer people to an appropriate facility where they can get the treatment they need.

The next most common excuse is probably fear of pain. Usually when I have a patient with severe dental phobia, it is because he or she had a childhood experience where they weren't treated properly. And, really, when that is the case, there's not a whole lot we can do to convince them otherwise, because those emotions are buried in their limbic system, or reptilian brain. You can go on and on about all the logical reasons they have no reason to feel that way, but that is exactly why phobias are described as irrational fears. Logic and reason reside in a different part of the brain—that's the cerebrum, the cerebral cortex. So, you cannot use logic to erase those patterns that are so deeply embedded; they will just occur, like a reflex reaction to the white coat, the smells, the sounds of the drill.

All I can do is to respect them and say, "I'm so sorry you had that experience. In this office, I assure you, things will be different. Your mouth is part of your body, and what you say, goes. If you need for me to stop, I'll stop. If you need to take a break, we'll take a break. One way or the other, we'll get the work done, but I'll make sure you're comfortable throughout the procedure." I actually said this to a ten-year-old girl named Meghan who was terribly afraid and was practically curling up in the fetal position right there in the dental chair. This was years ago, and I didn't see her for a long time after she graduated from high school. Then one day she came in for a cleaning visit and checkup while she was in town visiting her family. She reminded me about that conversation (which I had totally forgotten) and said it influenced her to study sociology and that she was now counseling battered women.

Even for those with the most extreme dental phobia, the good news is that with sedation dentistry, we have options. With oral sedatives or laughing gas, or simply using very gentle dentistry, fearful patents can come around, and they usually get better with each exposure to gentle care. And if not, there's always IV sedation, where they can be put completely under, and when they wake up their teeth are fixed. So, the pain issue is not supported either. In the modern office, we have lots of ways around that.

You can see a compendium of the five most common excuses not to see your dentist, and how to get over them, in the Tips and Takeaways section at the end of this chapter.

WE'RE ALL IN THIS TOGETHER

There are many ways to be more proactive about your health in general, and your dental health specifically. We have discussed most of them in this book, and I hope you take charge by enacting as many of them as can suit your lifestyle. But, I think that if there is one core that runs through all of what it takes to have a happy, healthy smile for life, it is developing a more positive attitude about dentistry, and your dentist.

With very few exceptions, nobody wakes up in the morning, jumps out of bed and is excited about going to see their dentist—I get that. But, I'd like to believe that I have designed my practice around giving my patients the most positive experience that any person could possibly have in a dental visit.

I realize that most people come in here dreading the bad news that they think they are going to get. So, I try to emphasize the positive from the outset. Most of the time, the very first thing we do is take an X-ray, and I will show that to them, and even if I see problems, I'll point out some good stuff first: "Oh you've got great bone level" or "Your jaw joint looks awesome." That sort of thing. This way, they don't get off to a negative start.

I also make it a point to meet with patients for an hour and a half on their first visit. I know that most people go to see the hygienist for an hour and only get to meet the dentist for maybe ten minutes. But we spend an hour and a half, one on one. We go over a lot of what we've discussed in this book, discussing nutrition, oral hygiene, and such. I tell them that most likely they will have their teeth cleaned twice a year. That means the other 363 days a year are on them, and they need to know what they're doing. So that hour and a half is for coaching, encouraging, informing. If there is work to be done, I tell them what their options are and let them make an informed decision. If they choose to do treatment, great—I'd love to be the dentist that does it for them. If they choose not to do it at this time, also great—I'd like to keep them in a healthy holding pattern so that they can choose that option later. I do think this approach is one of the main things that makes our practice unique.

I think health care in general has devolved quite a bit. To get into everything that is wrong with the state of health care today would likely take a whole other book. But in the context of what we've discussed in this book, I think the biggest problem is that most of us have let go of our own responsibility to ourselves—to keep ourselves healthy and happy. You've probably heard it said before that people can be like sheep, just going along with the flow. And there is an unfortunate general consensus out there that everybody's got health issues, so I might as well join the crowd. I think complacency is a big component of that.

Specific to dental health, in a lot of patients, that general sense of complacency gets combined with low expectations because they've come from a family background where parents had oral problems, and they just accept that they're going to be stuck with bad teeth because mom and dad had bad teeth. Or they present with severe dental anxiety—maybe they had a bad experience in another dental office as a child and they can't quite overcome their fear about reenacting that experience. All of these factors combine to result in an unfortunate number of people with poor smiles who convince themselves that "there's nothing I can do about it."

I hope that if you have read to this point you have come to realize that it doesn't have to be that way. Sometimes it can take a little work, sometimes it can take a lot. But I feel that, working together, I can get any patient to what I like to call the neutral zone, where often they can go for twenty years or more without any cavities, without any problems, without any aging of their teeth.

As you read these last words and close this book, my goal is that you breathe a deep sigh and realize that you can take charge of your own dental health. You can accept responsibility, and you can keep your teeth for a lifetime, comfortably and confidently. But I also hope that you realize you don't have to do it alone … we're partners, and we're all in this together.

TIPS AND TAKEAWAYS

THE TOP FIVE MOST COMMON OBJECTIONS
TO SEEING YOUR DENTIST

Excuse 1: It's too expensive

Reality:

- Early intervention saves money.

- Proper diet and proactive home care saves money.

- Wearing a protective mouth guard for some sports saves money.

- Avoiding dental care because of perceived cost generally leads to more expensive treatments.

- Many payment plans are available to those with good credit ratings.

- Most treatment can be phased, spreading costs over time.

Excuse 2: Dental phobia

Reality:

- General anxiety—We can eliminate sounds with music via earbuds, and avoid bad memory-triggering smells by using natural versus chemical cleaning products, an oxygen mask, or essential oils (peppermint, lemon, lavender) just above the lip.

- Pain and discomfort—Nobody loves dental injections, but we use a technique that pre-numbs before the actual injection that has been very popular with our patients. We can also use laughing gas, or IV, or oral sedation.

Excuse 3: I don't want my teeth altered

Reality:

- Most dental procedures actually alter natural teeth very little. Depending on the procedure, the enamel is reduced by only 0.3–1.0 millimeters on the vertical surfaces of the teeth and 1.5–2.0 millimeters on the biting surfaces, in order to create room for the porcelain. For reference, a typical credit card is 1 millimeter thick. The reduction is taken from the desired endpoint, so if the teeth are worn, or eroded, we may actually have to add material to the tooth to get the desired endpoint.

Excuse 4: I'm too busy

Reality:

- Even dentists have to go to the dentist. I arrange my work schedule so that I can take a longer lunch or an afternoon off, or start later in the morning. I do the same with doctor appointments, eye exams, etc. You simply need to plan ahead and make time in your schedule to attend to good health.

- We respect our patients' time. We strive to run on schedule (about 98 percent of the time) and let patients know how long they can expect to be in the office.

Excuse 5: I will not like the result

Reality:

- In our office, the case is not complete until the patient is happy with the result. We can make this claim because our design phase incorporates the patient's desires with a planned outcome.

- Photography allows good communication between the patient, doctor, and lab technicians.

- Temporary crowns or veneers can be verified for speech and esthetics, then copied in the lab phase.

- Choices about translucency, color, shape, and texture are discussed early in treatment in order to exceed the patient's expectations.

EIGHT QUESTIONS TO ASK YOUR DENTIST

1. How much will it cost?

Fees are based on a number of factors, including overhead (facility, equipment, etc.), complexity of the process, materials used, and experience of the team. A well-known and highly respected lab technician will command a higher fee than an entry-level technician in a developing nation. This is a situation where you don't want to pay too little. Paying for quality that lasts and results that meet or exceed your expectations, as well as having a relatively pleasant experience throughout the process, will be worth so much more over the years than paying less initially, having a bad experience, and being unhappy with the results.

2. How many of these procedures has the dentist performed?

Experience matters. Proficiency comes from doing something over and over again. Just like with musicians, performance improves with practice. Young dentists may be quite adept at performing a particular procedure, and mature dentists may be trying a new procedure for the first time. It pays to ask.

3. What assurance do I have that I will be pleased with the result?

I recently saw a new patient who had just had four veneers placed on her front teeth. They looked terrible! She was so traumatized by the long process, the discomfort, and the disappointing result that she had no intention of returning to the dentist who did the work. Only when she saw the final results and expressed her dissatisfaction did she find out that the office policy was no refunds or discounts. In our office, we work with the patient through the design and try-in process and validate satisfaction with the temporaries before instructing the lab technician to copy those temporary restorations for the length, shape, and position of the final restorations. We aren't finished until you are happy.

4. What materials will you use for my dental work?

While you may assume that your new fillings are going to be tooth colored, some dentists still like to use silver amalgam filling material. You may be expecting all-ceramic crowns, only to find the ones you received are gold. Again, if your dentist doesn't bring up the conversation about what your desired outcome is, you should ask.

5. How long will my appointment take?

Some offices run faster and some run slower. Higher-volume clinics will see more patients and delegate more of the work to auxiliary personnel while the dentist sees other patients. Lower-volume practices, like mine, enable the dentist to stay with the patient, delegate less, and likely shorten your time in the chair.

6. How long before my restorations come back from the lab?

Return times on lab work vary greatly, usually between two to six weeks. While you may think faster is better, sometimes we want to allow time for tissues to heal or for the bite to stabilize, so more waiting time is actually better. It shouldn't be a problem when you have beautiful, secure temporary restorations in the interim.

7. Will it hurt?

Procedures for crowns, veneers, and fillings generally don't have much, if any, accompanying pain, and over-the-counter painkillers are fine for any tenderness you may experience. Other procedures, such as bone or soft-tissue grafts, can require prescription painkillers for a few days, and up to a week. Be sure to ask before you schedule your dental appointment the day before going on vacation!

8. What if there's a problem?

Problems can, and do, arise from time to time. Crowns (final or temporary) can come off, teeth can be sensitive; the bite may need adjustment. In my office, we call patients after any procedure that involves numbing and check to see that they are feeling okay. We see emergencies promptly and make appropriate referrals to specialists when needed. If problems occur at other times, such as weekends or holidays, there is always someone on call to help out.

CONCLUSION

Years ago, I had the opportunity to obtain a pilot's license after taking flying lessons out of a small airport near my neighborhood. I would rent one of the flying school's small Cessna airplanes and take off for an excursion over rolling fields and winding streams west of Houston that were still a safe distance from busy metropolitan airports. Takeoffs were exhilarating, and after working on tiny teeth in confined spaces all week long, it was a liberating feeling being up in the sky.

After a time, I would venture out on longer flights—to Waco, Austin, or Galveston. By flying above the traffic and stop signs, I found I could reach my destination in about half the time of driving a car, even counting the time it took to log a flight plan and conduct a preflight check. That's what I was thinking when my sister, Marcia, came to Texas from Colorado to visit my parents in Longview, about a four-hour drive from my home. By flying, I could make it to East Texas in time for lunch and a visit and be back home in Houston in time for dinner.

The morning of my flight was humid and balmy, but the weather forecast indicated there would be good conditions all day for my VFR trip (visual flight rating, meaning I could see the ground below). I logged my flight plan and took off to the north.

While you're flying, you don't notice tailwinds and headwinds all that much, other than the way they may affect your speed—tailwinds speed you up, headwinds slow you down. But you do notice a crosswind, because you have to angle the plane in order to stay on your desired course. It's when you land that the crosswind becomes a challenge. So with my family on the ground at my destination airport, watching me come in for the world's bumpiest one-wheel landing, I made it safely to East Texas in time for lunch at a nearby restaurant.

It was through the restaurant windows that I noticed the trees bending over in the increasingly strong winds, and I became concerned about my trip home. A front was coming in from the north, pushing the balmy weather toward the coast, but right now, flags were flapping in the breeze and debris was whirling in small dust devils.

Back at the airport, I called flight services and they told me that two small planes had gone down in the area and I should stay on the ground. I agreed! I called the flight school that had leased the plane to me and told them I was keeping their plane overnight and would return it the next day, assuming weather conditions allowed.

The next morning, weather conditions were perfect. The front had gone through during the night, bringing in clear, cool weather along with a tailwind for my flight home. I borrowed a sweater from my mother, cranked up the heat in the plane, and took off.

Perhaps thirty or forty minutes into my flight, I started to feel strange, like I'd had a couple of glasses of wine. I was dizzy and sleepy. I could barely stay awake. Just then, I remembered a written question on a flight test and realized there must be carbon monoxide coming into the cabin from the exhaust system. Fighting the fatigue, I turned the heater off, trimmed the plane to slowly climb in altitude, and opened the side window. And then—I totally blacked out.

After a time, my thoughts returned, but my body couldn't respond. "Open your eyes," I told myself. "I can't," a voice inside my head replied. "Lift your head!" But my head wouldn't lift, at least not at first. As the fresh air circulated in the cabin, I was able to raise my head and look around. I'm still not sure how long I was out—maybe twenty or thirty minutes based on my new location. The winds had pushed me toward Houston, but I was nearly over Lake Conroe, heading straight into airspace controlled by Houston Intercontinental Airport, later named after George H.W. Bush. I had awakened just in time to make appropriate corrections and redirect my flight path to land at my neighborhood airport. I'm not ashamed to admit that I literally kneeled on the ground after getting out of the plane and uttered a prayer of gratitude for my life. Apparently, it was not my day to die.

When you have a life-changing moment like the one I experienced, it changes your perspective about life forever. Every day is a gift from God, and I want to savor every aspect of it. I want to relish the sights, sounds, and flavors of each experience. I choose to forgive others when they say and do hurtful things and to find the positive aspect of challenges.

And most of all, I want to assist others, to help them get more out of life. Offering patients an engaging—and many actually say an enjoyable—experience obtaining true dental health and beauty is the most impactful way I am able to do this. Perhaps angels flew that airplane that day while I was unconscious in order to give me the chance to fulfill my purpose of enriching the lives of others through this amazing career I've had the privilege of enjoying for over thirty years.

CPSIA information can be obtained
at www.ICGtesting.com
Printed in the USA
BVHW091136231218
536277BV00013B/316/P